Some G.I. Diet Success Stories

"I started the G.I. Diet at the beginning of March 2004 . . . It is now four months later and I'm 25 pounds lighter. I feel stronger, have more energy and am fitting into clothes that haven't fit in ages! . . . For once in my life I actually believe I can get to my goal weight . . . Thank you for such a wonderful, healthy way of eating that WORKS!" **Alicia**

"I lost 85 pounds in 22 weeks . . . There is certainly no more rewarding personal journey than transforming your body into what you always wanted it to be. I can't begin to express how valuable the G.I. Diet has been to making this happen." **Derek**

"My husband is down 40 pounds and I'm down 20 pounds!! The G.I. Diet rocks!! We're never hungry, we can't believe the gradual and constant weight loss, and we can't believe that we can eat out, travel, celebrate special events and still, albeit sometimes partially, stick to the regime and keep the weight off. I've spent the last two days taking my husband's pants, shorts and shirts in. Some of them by 4½ inches! He's a happy guy and I'm the happy girl who can reach all the way around him and hug him to death." **Joann**

"I'm thrilled with the results I've had so far. I, or rather my family, which includes my husband and my two sons, began eating the G.I. way at the beginning of September. As of October 22, I had lost 14 pounds . . . Can you believe that since I started eating better and my colleagues took notice of my weight loss and energy, four others have joined what we call our 'G.I. Jane Club'?" **Mary**

"I started living the G.I. Diet three months ago and have shed 43 pounds and 6 inches off my waistline . . . I follow the program religiously and have made up my mind to eat like this for the rest of my life. I used to be a junk food addict but now even the smell of junk food turns my stomach. Thanks again for your program. It was literally a life saver." **Ray**

"After many different attempts at losing weight, I finally found success with the G.I. Diet! I started in early March and have already lost 15 pounds. I'm 55 years old, and after trying other weight loss plans, I'd just about surrendered to the women's 'middle-age weight gain' theory. But with the G.I. Diet, the pounds and inches melt away. I'm wearing clothes I haven't worn in years and my energy level is unbelievable. No more mid-afternoon slumps!" **Jan**

"I cannot believe the results of this diet. I am thirty-six years old and have had a weight problem all my life. This is the first diet that I can actually do for longer than one month (I am on the sixth week), and that keeps providing results. I have lost about fifteen pounds, but it is not the weight loss that I am impressed with but rather how I feel. I feel great!" **Toni**

"Lost 40+ pounds in a matter of 2+ months (from 210 lbs. to 170 lbs.). No more headaches! Blood pressure back down from 180/120 to normal reading. My doctor can't believe the change. Best I've felt in years." **Joe**

Praise from the Professionals

"The G.I. Diet is an innovative, realistic, uncomplicated long-term approach to successful weight management. It presents the reader with a simple guide to food choices, both at home and away, with easy-to-remember images, practical tips, tasty recipes and strategies for feedback and self-monitoring." **Dr. Michael J. Sole, BSc. (Hon), MD, FRCP(C), FACC, FAHA**

"For the management of diabetes, the most effective amongst the current crop of diets is the glycemic index (G.I.) diet. . . . The G.I. approach postulated by Gallop is particularly good because it's easy to understand and apply to everyday life." **Dr. Medeve in** *Diabetes Dialogue* **(Canadian Diabetes Association)**

"Most diet books are too wordy, their plans too complicated and their quick-fix promises filled with false hope. Rick Gallop's G.I. Diet is based on solid science but is easy to access. If you can understand a stop light, you can lose weight on this amazing diet—eating your favourite green-light foods all the way." **Marilyn Linton,** *Toronto Sun* **health columnist**

"An excellent guide for people looking to reduce their risk of cardiovascular disease. The G.I. Diet reflects Gallop's highly successful years as president and CEO of the Heart and Stroke Foundation of Ontario, working at the interface of real world problems and disease." **Dr. David Jenkins, MD, PhD., DSc., Professor, Department of Nutritional Sciences, Faculty of Medicine, University of Toronto**

"This book is timely, with increasing obesity across the developed and parts of the developing world, and together with advice from the New Food Pyramid could well lessen the epidemic of obesity-related illness and death from diabetes and heart and blood vessel disease worldwide. I use this book in my writings and discussions on health internationally, and in my practice, with feedback that is easy to use, simplifies a complex subject, and it works."
Dr. Vivian S. Rambihar, Cardiologist, Toronto

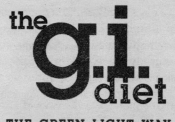

the g.i. diet

THE GREEN-LIGHT WAY
TO PERMANENT WEIGHT LOSS

REVISED AND UPDATED

RICK GALLOP

Past President of the Heart & Stroke Foundation of Ontario

SEAL BOOKS

THE REVISED G.I. DIET
Seal Books/published by arrangement with
    Random House Canada
Random House Canada edition published 2005
Seal Books edition published January 2006

ISBN-13: 978-0-7704-2994-2
ISBN-10: 0-7704-2994-7

Interior design: Jean Lightfoot Peters

Seal Books are published by
Random House of Canada Limited.
"Seal Books" and the portrayal of a seal are the property of
Random House of Canada Limited.

Visit Random House of Canada Limited's website:
www.randomhouse.ca

PRINTED AND BOUND IN THE USA

OPM 10 9 8 7 6 5 4 3 2

Contents

Foreword by Dr. Michael J. Sole viii

Introduction 1

CHAPTER ONE The Problem 4

CHAPTER TWO How Much Weight Should I Lose? 23

CHAPTER THREE Phase I 33

CHAPTER FOUR Ready, Set, Go! 70

CHAPTER FIVE The Green-Light Glossary 77

CHAPTER SIX Meal Ideas 85

CHAPTER SEVEN Phase II 108

CHAPTER EIGHT Recipes 115

CHAPTER NINE Exercise 200

CHAPTER TEN Health 216

CHAPTER ELEVEN Supplements 223

Appendices 228

Acknowledgements 244

Index 246

Recipe Index 255

Foreword

It's hard to ignore, especially as a cardiologist, the fact that obesity has ballooned into a crisis of epidemic proportions in North America. It affects one in three adults and one in four children and teenagers. In my own practice, I see a disproportionate number of patients who are overweight or obese, as obesity is a recognized risk factor for conditions that are the foundations for heart attack and stroke. Contrary to popular belief, abdominal fat is not merely a passive repository of excess weight; it is actively associated with hormones that endanger health. A waist circumference of greater than 40 inches for men and 35 inches for women is associated with a high-risk profile for coronary heart disease.

Millions of people are on diets, spending billions of dollars on self-help, quick-fix books, weight loss programs, diet drinks and foods. The continued growth of the weight loss industry is assured since so many of these plans and practices fail in the face of unachievable expectations. Indeed, many dieters rebound to weights exceeding their original. Obesity is a chronic condition, and effective weight management requires a long-term behavioural strategy. The promises of easy weight loss diets are false and will not result in long-term success. The marked early weight loss seen in low carbohydrate diets, for example, is due to water loss with depletion of carbohydrate (glycogen) stores, not fat loss. Low carbohydrate diets are high in protein and fat and low in fibre and several important micronutrients; thus they provide no basis for long-term healthful eating and permanent maintenance of weight loss. These diets are associated with an increase in constipation and headache, and there is concern in the medical community that they pose an increased risk of cardiovascular disease and cancer.

The typical dieter is doomed to repeat failure because he or she chases the fantasy of a dream weight and a fast solution rather than learns from experience and finally confronts the reality of achievable, permanent weight loss. The laws of thermodynamics are irrefutable, even for dieters: to lose one pound of fat you must achieve a deficit of 3,600 calories.

Why read *The G.I. Diet*, another book on a long shelf of "New You" promises? If you want weight loss fiction, this book isn't for you. *The G.I. Diet* is an innovative, realistic, uncomplicated, long-term approach to successful weight management. To create this diet, Rick Gallop has drawn on his long experience with the Heart and Stroke Foundation of Ontario and its research and public education programs. He discusses the principles of nutrition and illustrates these with anecdotes and humour, which bring them alive and make them easy to digest.

Building on this practical knowledge, Rick then tackles the problem of weight loss as a long-term issue, leading you through the supportive elements of behavioural change, including the development of achievable specific goals: How much should I lose per week? Exactly how will I do it? If I fail one day, how do I respond? How do I cope with breakfast meetings, luncheon meetings, muffins in midday meetings, and then fast-food dinners or more formal dinners out? You only live once and food is one of life's great pleasures. Counting calories is not a preferred option.

The G.I. Diet presents the reader with a simple guide to food choices, both at home and away, with easy-to-remember images, practical tips, tasty recipes and strategies for feedback and self-monitoring. The critical importance of exercise is also addressed. Finally, Rick Gallop has included an assortment of self-help weight loss tools—additions that the reader is certain to find useful.

With a heavy travel schedule, lunchtime meetings and dinners out, I must be continually vigilant about my weight. The principles and ideas described by Rick Gallop in this book have certainly been beneficial to me. *The G.I. Diet* charts a course that if followed will deliver its promise of permanent weight loss.

Michael J. Sole, BSC (Hon), MD, FRCP(C), FACC, FAHA
Former Chief of Cardiology, University Health Network
Professor of Medicine and Physiology
Founder of The Heart and Stroke, Richard Lewar Centre of Excellence, University of Toronto

Introduction

I am so amazed and delighted by the number of people who have picked up *The G.I. Diet*, followed its advice and slimmed down to their ideal weight. In a world of fad diets and bad advice, hundreds of thousands of people have chosen the best and healthiest way to permanent weight loss—hooray! The book has become a national bestseller in Canada, the United States and Britain and is now available in over a dozen countries in ten languages. And every day I receive readers' letters and e-mails telling me how much weight they've lost and how it's changed their lives. This truly has been my greatest reward and satisfaction, because this is exactly what I set out to do when I first wrote the book: to help people get healthy and feel good about themselves.

I know what it's like to be overweight and to try one deprivation diet after another with no success. Several years ago, as a result of a lower back disc problem, I had to give up my regular morning jog. Well, it didn't take long for me to gain 22 pounds and—even worse for my vanity—4 inches on my waist. As president of the Heart and

Stroke Foundation of Ontario, my job was to raise funds for research into heart disease and stroke and to promote healthy lifestyle choices to reduce people's risk for those diseases. And there I was, overweight myself! All of a sudden I had to practise what I had been preaching for ten years—a sobering experience. I tried about a dozen different leading diets, calculated calories, points, carbs and blocks, suffered hunger pangs, hallucinated about food, and never managed to lose those 22 pounds.

Luckily, when I was just about at the end of my rope, I happened upon a way of eating that changed my life. I finally lost the weight that had been plaguing me for so long, and it was a revelation. You can imagine how excited I was; I wanted to tell everyone about it, end their dieting frustrations forever and lower their risk for heart attack and stroke. I asked fifty volunteers to try my new-found weight loss solution. But after one year, only two of those volunteers had managed to stick to the diet. I was completely floored. I interviewed every one of the forty-eight volunteers to find out why they had dropped out. Everyone gave the same two reasons: 1) They felt hungry and deprived while on the diet; and 2) They hated having to count and measure calories, points and carbs. I realized that if I could eliminate those two obstacles, namely hunger and complexity, the diet would work for everyone.

The result was *The G.I. Diet*, and the question of whether it works has been answered by the tens of thousands of e-mails I've received. The overwhelming response encouraged me to write *Living the G.I. Diet*, which gives more tips on how to stick to the diet as well as over one hundred G.I. recipes from Emily Richards, the popular TV co-host of *Canadian Living Cooks*.

Since the publication of the books, more and more research has been done on the effectiveness of a low-G.I. diet. Recently, a Harvard study showed that in animal trials, those fed a balanced diet with high-G.I. carbohydrates gained more weight, doubled their body fat, and lost more muscle mass than those fed an identical diet with low-G.I. carbohydrates. The high-G.I. group also saw an increase in their blood sugar and a high likelihood of developing diabetes.

With all the new research and information coming in, I decided to write this new revised and updated edition. It includes new additions to the red-, yellow- and green-light food listings, forty new recipes, a meal planner and a host of personal stories to help motivate you with your own weight loss goals. I look forward to receiving your comments and suggestions through my Web site, www.gidiet.com.

The greatest dream in life is to feel you have made a difference to someone. I'd like to express my appreciation to those hundreds of thousands of readers who have made this dream come true for me!

CHAPTER ONE

The Problem

While I was waging my personal battle of the bulge, I couldn't help but be struck by the number of people who were engaged in the same struggle. The statistics are truly astonishing: 50 percent of Canadian adults today are overweight. That's more than double what it was only ten years ago. Even more worrying is the tripling of the obesity rate among children over the past twenty years. What's happened to us? Why have we gained so much weight in recent years?

The simple explanation is that people are eating too many calories. Unless one denies the basic laws of thermodynamics, the equation never changes: consume more calories than you expend and the surplus is stored in the body as fat. That's the inescapable fact. But that doesn't explain why people today are eating more calories than they used to. To answer that question we must first understand the three key components of any diet—carbohydrates, fats and proteins—and how they work in our digestive system. Since fats are probably the least understood part, let's start with them.

Fats

Fat is definitely a bad word these days, and it engenders an enormous amount of confusion and contradiction. But are you aware that fats are absolutely essential for a nutritious diet? They contain various key elements that are crucial to the digestive process.

The next fact might also surprise you: fat does not necessarily make you fat. The quantity you consume does. And that's something that's often difficult to control, because your body *loves* fat. Non-fat foods require lots of processing to be transformed into those fat cells around your waist and hips; fatty foods just slide right in. Processing takes energy, and your body hates wasting energy. It needs to expend about 20 to 25 percent of the energy it gets from a non-fat food just to process it. So your body definitely prefers fat, and as we all know from personal experience, it will do everything it can to persuade us to eat more of it. That's why fatty foods like juicy steaks, chocolate, and decadent ice creams taste so good to us. But because fat contains twice as many calories per gram as carbohydrates and proteins, we really have to be careful about the amount of fat we eat.

In addition to limiting *how much* fat we consume, we must also pay attention to the *type* of fat. While the type of fat has no effect on our weight, it is critical to our health—especially heart health.

There are four types of fat: the best, the better, the bad and the really ugly. The "bad" fats are called saturated fats, and they are easily recognizable because they almost always come from animal sources and they solidify at room temperature. Butter, cheese and meat are all high in saturated fats. There are a couple of others you should be aware of too: coconut oil and palm oil are two vegetable oils that are saturated, and because they are cheap, they are used in many snack foods, especially cookies. Saturated fats are a principal cause of heart disease because they boost cholesterol, which in turn thickens arteries and causes heart attack and stroke. And recent research has demonstrated that several cancers—breast, colon and prostate—as well as Alzheimer's are associated with diets high in saturated fat.

Fifteen years ago a wealthy American industrialist had a heart attack. Like many successful businessmen he hated surprises, and he wanted to know what had caused the unexpected turn in his health. When he discovered that many leading food products contain tropical oils such as palm and coconut, he took out a full-page ad in *The Wall Street Journal* declaring: "THESE 9 PRODUCTS ARE KILLING AMERICANS." Within forty-eight hours, eight of the nine products were reformulated without the tropical oils. Check your labels.

The "really ugly" fats are potentially the most dangerous. They are vegetable oils that have been heat-treated to make them thicken. These hydrogenated oils take on the worst characteristics of saturated fats, so don't use them, and avoid snack foods, baked goods and cereals that contain them. Check the label for "hydrogenated oils," "partially hydrogenated oils" or "trans fat."

The "better" fats are called polyunsaturated, and they are cholesterol free. Most vegetable oils, such as corn and sunflower, fall into this category. What you should really be using, however, are monounsaturated fats, the "best," which are found in olives, peanuts, almonds, and olive and canola oils. Monounsaturated fats have a beneficial effect on cholesterol and are good for your heart. (See chapter 10 for more information on cholesterol and heart disease.) Though fancy olive oils are expensive, you can get the same health benefits from reasonably priced house brands at your supermarket. Olive oil is used extensively in the famed Mediterranean diet, which is also rich in fruits and vegetables. Because of their diet, southern Europeans have some of the lowest rates of heart disease in the world, and obesity is not a problem in those countries. So look for monounsaturated fats and oils on food labels. Most manufacturers who use them will say so, because they know it's a key selling point for informed consumers.

Another highly beneficial oil, which is in a category of its own, contains a wonderful ingredient called omega-3. This oil is found in deep-sea fish such as salmon and in flax and canola seed. It's extremely good for your heart health (see page 227).

So we know that it's important to avoid the bad and the really ugly fats and to incorporate the best fats in our diets to make our hearts healthy. Many of us have tried to lower our fat intake by using leaner cuts of meat and drinking lower-fat milk. But even with these modifications our fat consumption hasn't decreased. Why? Because many of our favourite foods—like crackers, muffins, cereals and fast foods—contain hidden fats. Detecting them often seems to require an advanced degree in nutrition, since labelling of nutritional components has until recently been voluntary in Canada (unlike the U.S.). A good rule of thumb is to avoid any food whose package does not list its nutritional components; this usually means that the manufacturer has something to hide.

COOKING OILS/FATS

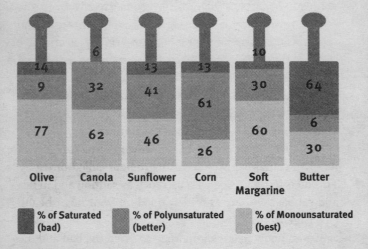

% of Saturated (bad)	% of Polyunsaturated (better)	% of Monounsaturated (best)

So we're not eating less fat, but contrary to popular belief, neither are we eating more. Fat consumption in this country has remained virtually constant over the past ten years, while obesity numbers have doubled. Obviously, fat isn't the culprit. What has increased is our consumption of *grain*. Grain is a carbohydrate, so let's look at how carbohydrates work.

TO SUM UP:
1. Eat less fat overall and look for low-fat alternatives to your current diet.
2. Eat monounsaturated and polyunsaturated fats only.

Dear Mr. Gallop,

I would like to express my sincere thanks for *The G.I. Diet*, as so many other indebted "bulge fighters" have done . . . After 140 days on the diet I am down 20 pounds, and 7 inches off my waist. But this is not the best part—I've done this before. This time the weight came off painlessly, and with the assurance that I have a lifelong, effective and healthy way to control my weight. In addition, I have increased energy . . . I really think that as a public service, Health Canada should endorse and promote *The G.I. Diet*.

Thanks again,

Gilles

Carbohydrates

Unfortunately there is a great deal of misinformation in the marketplace about carbohydrates. Much of it stems from the current low-carb diet fad, which would have you believe that if you stick to low-carb foods, you'll lose weight. If only it were that simple. The reality is that you need carbs for a healthy diet and you shouldn't avoid them. The key is to choose the right, or good, carbs, like fruit, vegetables, legumes, whole grains, nuts and low-fat dairy products. These foods are the primary source of energy for your body, which converts them into glucose. The glucose dissolves in your bloodstream and is diverted to those parts of your body that use energy, like your muscles and your brain. (It may surprise you to know that when you are resting your brain uses about two-thirds of the glucose in your system!)

Carbohydrates, therefore, are essential for your body to function. They are rich in fibre, vitamins and minerals, including antioxidants, which we now believe play a critical role in protecting against disease, especially heart disease and cancer. For years we've been advised by doctors, nutritionists and government to eat a low-fat, high-carbohydrate diet, and grains form the base of Canada's Food Guide. The trouble with this is that it has encouraged us all to rely too much on them. Just look at the amount of space dedicated to grain-based products in our supermarkets today: huge cracker, cookie and snack food sections; whole aisles of cereals; numerous shelves of pastas and noodles; and baskets and baskets of bagels, rolls, muffins and loaves of bread. I can remember when bagels were exclusive to the Jewish community; now most food stores carry half a dozen different varieties, and chains of bagel stores are spread across the country. Muffins were never as abundant as they are today. (Not so very long ago, a colleague of mine was coming in to work bleary-eyed every day. When I asked her what was happening, she explained that she was staying up each night baking different flavoured muffins for a new retail idea of her husband, Michael Bregman. He went on to found the mmmuffins chain— and the rest, as they say, is history.)

GRAIN CONSUMPTION (pounds per capita)

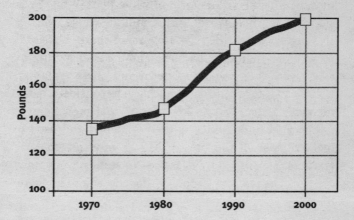

Source: U.S. Department of Agriculture (1970–2000)

Another modern food sensation has been pasta, once viewed as an ethnic specialty in North America. That's hard to believe today, with pasta a staple on most restaurant menus and every family's shopping list. Eighty percent of Canadian homes now serve pasta at least once a week. And our snack-food options have multiplied: crackers, tortilla chips, corn chips, pretzels and countless varieties of cookies, to name just a few.

In 1970 the average North American ate about 135 pounds of grain. By 2000 that figure had risen to about 200 pounds. That's a 50-percent increase! Why should we be concerned about this? Aren't wheat, corn and rice low-fat? How could grain be making us fat?

The answer lies in the *type* of grain we're eating today, most of which is in the form of white flour. White flour starts off as whole wheat. At the mill the whole wheat is steamed and scarified by tiny razor-sharp blades to remove the bran, or outer shell, and the endosperm, the next layer. Then the wheat germ and oil are removed because they turn rancid too quickly to be considered commercially viable. What's left after all that processing is unbleached flour, which is then whitened and used to make almost all the breads, bagels, muffins, cookies, crackers, cereals and pastas we consume. Even many "brown" breads are simply artificially coloured white bread.

It's not just grain that's highly processed nowadays. A hundred years ago most of the food people ate came straight from the farm to the dinner table. Lack of refrigeration and scant knowledge of food chemistry meant that most food remained in its original state. However, advances in science, along with the migration of many women out of the kitchen and into the workforce, led to a revolution in prepared foods. Everything became geared to speed and simplicity of preparation. Today's high-speed flour mills use steel rollers rather than the traditional grinding stones to produce an extraordinarily finely ground product, ideal for producing light and fluffy breads and pastries. We now have instant rice and potatoes, as well as entire meals that are ready to eat after just a few minutes in the microwave.

The problem with all this is that the more a food is processed beyond its natural state, the less processing your body has to do to digest it. And the quicker you digest your food, the sooner you are hungry again, and the more you tend to eat. We all know the difference between eating a bowl of old-fashioned slow-cooking oatmeal and a bowl of sugary cold cereal. The oatmeal stays with you—it "sticks to your ribs" as my mother used to say—whereas you are looking for your next meal an hour after eating the bowl of sugary cereal. That's why our ancestors did not have the obesity problem we have today; their foods were basically unprocessed and natural. All the great food companies, like Kraft, General Foods, Kellogg's, McCain, Nabisco and Del Monte, only started processing and packaging natural foods in the past century or so.

Our fundamental problem, then, is that we are eating foods that are too easily digested by our bodies. Clearly, we can't wind back the clock to simpler times, but we need somehow to slow down the digestive process so we feel hungry less often. How can we do that? Well, we have to eat foods that are "slow-release," that break down at a slow and steady rate in our digestive system, leaving us feeling fuller for longer.

How do we identify those "slow-release" foods? There are two clues. The first is the amount of fibre in the food. Fibre, in simple terms, provides low-calorie filler. It does double duty, in fact: it literally fills up your stomach, so you feel satiated; and your body takes much longer to break it down, so it stays with you longer and slows down the digestive process. There are two forms of fibre: soluble and insoluble. Soluble fibre is found in foods like oatmeal, beans, barley and citrus fruits, and has been shown to lower blood cholesterol levels. Insoluble fibre is important for normal bowel function and is typically found in whole wheat breads and cereals and most vegetables.

The second tool in identifying slow-release foods is the glycemic index, which I will now explain. It is the core of this diet and the key to successful weight management.

TO SUM UP:
Eat foods that have not been highly processed and that do not contain highly processed ingredients.

The Glycemic Index

The glycemic index measures the speed at which you digest food and convert it to glucose, your body's energy source. The faster the food breaks down, the higher the rating on the index. The index sets sugar (glucose) at 100 and scores all foods against that number. Here are some examples:

Baguette	95	Donut	76	Muffin (bran)	56	Oatmeal	42	Fettuccine	32
Instant Rice	87	Cheerios	75	Popcorn low-fat	55	Spagetti	41	Beans	31
Baked Potatoes	84	Bagel	72	Orange	44	Apple	38	Grapefruit	25
Cornflakes	84	Raisins	64	All-Bran	43	Tomato	38	Fat- and sugar-free Yogurt	14

The chart on the next page illustrates the impact of sugar on the level of glucose in your bloodstream compared with kidney beans, which have a low G.I. rating. As you can see, there is a dramatic difference between the two. Sugar is quickly converted into glucose, which dissolves in your bloodstream, spiking its glucose level. It also disappears quickly, leaving you wanting more. Have you ever eaten a large Chinese meal, with lots of noodles and rice, only to find yourself hungry again an hour or two later? That's because your body rapidly converted the rice and noodles, high-G.I. foods, to glucose, which then quickly disappeared from your bloodstream. Something most of us experience regularly is the feeling of lethargy that follows an hour or so after a fast-food lunch, which generally consists of high-G.I. foods. The surge of glucose followed by the rapid drain leaves us starved of energy. So what do we do? Around mid-afternoon we look for a quick sugar fix, or snack, to bring us out of the slump. A few cookies or a bag of chips cause another rush of glucose, which disappears a short time later—and so the vicious cycle continues. No wonder we're a nation of snackers!

When you eat a high-G.I. food and experience a rapid spike in blood sugar, your pancreas releases the hormone insulin. Insulin does two things extremely well. First, it reduces the level of glucose in your bloodstream by

G.I. IMPACT ON SUGAR LEVELS

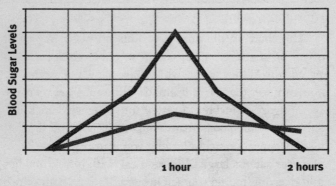

GI 100 Sugar (Glucose)   GI 27 Kidney beans

diverting it into various body tissues for immediate short-term use or by storing it as fat—which is why glucose disappears so quickly. Second, it inhibits the conversion of body fat back into glucose for the body to burn. This evolutionary feature is a throwback to the days when our ancestors were hunter-gatherers, habitually experiencing times of feast or famine. When food was in abundance, the body stored its surplus as fat to tide it over the inevitable days of famine. Insulin was the champion in this process, both helping to accumulate fat and then guarding its depletion.

Today, everything has changed except our stomachs. A digestive system that has taken millions of years to evolve is, in a comparative evolutionary blink of an eye, expected to cope with a food revolution. We don't have to hunt and search for food any more; we have a guaranteed supply of highly processed foods with a multitude of tempting flavours and textures at the supermarket. Not only are we consuming more easily digested calories, but we're not expending as much energy in finding our food and keeping ourselves warm—the two major preoccupations of our ancestors.

Since insulin is the key trigger to storing glucose as well as the sentry that keeps those fat cells intact, it is crucial to maintain low insulin levels when you are trying to lose weight, and that means avoiding high-G.I. foods. Low-G.I. foods such as apples are like the tortoise to the high-G.I. foods' hare. They break down in your digestive system at a slow, steady rate. You don't get a quick sugar fix when you eat them, but, tortoiselike, they stay the course, so that you feel full longer. Therefore if you want to lose weight, you must stick to low-G.I. foods.

But the fact that a food has a low G.I. does not necessarily make it desirable. The other critical factor determining whether a food will allow us to lose weight is its calorie content. It's the combination of low-G.I foods with few calories, i.e., low in sugar and fat, that is the "magic bullet" of the G.I. Diet. Low-G.I., low-calorie foods make you feel more satiated than do foods with a high G.I. and calorie level. Later in this book I will provide you with a comprehensive chart identifying the foods that will make you fat and those that will allow you to lose weight. Don't expect all the low-G.I. foods to be tasteless and boring! There are many delicious and satisfying choices that will make you feel as though you aren't even on a diet.

I've already mentioned two of the principal factors that contribute to a food's G.I. rating: the degree of processing it undergoes before it is digested and how much fibre it contains. But there are two other important components that inhibit the rapid breakdown of food in our digestive system, and they are fat and protein. The influence of these two factors can lead to some surprising, and confusing, results. Peanut butter, for example, has a low G.I. because of its high fat and protein content. Similarly, whole milk has a lower G.I. than skim, and fruitcake has a lower G.I. than melba toast. Fat, like fibre, acts as a brake in the digestive process. When combined with other foods it becomes a barrier to digestive juices. It also signals the brain that you are satisfied and do not require more food. But we know that many fats are harmful to your heart, and they contain twice the number of calories per gram as carbohydrates and protein. Since protein also acts as a brake in the digestive process, let's look at it in more detail.

TO SUM UP:

1. Low-G.I. foods are slower to digest, so you feel satiated longer.
2. Keeping insulin levels low inhibits the formation of fat and assists in the conversion of fat back into energy.
3. The key to losing weight is to eat low-G.I., low-calorie foods.

Hi Rick,

First, the biggest Thank You! . . . I have been following the G.I. Diet now for eight weeks and have lost 15 pounds. I read your book within a day and couldn't believe that I had struggled for fifteen years at various diet clubs and here in front of me was the obvious answer . . . The first week I couldn't believe I was losing weight—it didn't feel as if I was doing anything to reduce, yet I lost an astonishing 6 pounds! . . . You're my hero!

Jill

Protein

One-half of your dry body weight is made up of protein, i.e., your muscles, organs, skin and hair. Obviously protein is an essential part of your diet. It's required to build and repair body tissue, and figures in nearly all metabolic reactions.

Protein is also much more effective than carbohydrates or fat in satisfying hunger. It will make you feel fuller longer, which is why you should always try to incorporate some protein in every meal and snack. It will help keep you alert and feeling full. Again, however, the type of protein you consume is important. Proteins are found in a broad range of food products, both animal and vegetable, and not just in red meat and whole dairy products, which are high in saturated or "bad" fat.

So what sort of protein should you be including in your diet? Choose low-fat proteins: lean or low-fat cuts of meat that have been trimmed of any visible fat; skinless poultry; fresh, frozen or canned fish (but not the kind that's coated with batter, which is invariably high in fat); low-fat dairy products like skim milk (believe it or not, after a couple of weeks of drinking it, it tastes just like 2%); low-fat yogurt (look for the artificially sweetened versions, as many manufacturers pump up the sugar as they drop the fat) and low-fat cottage cheese; liquid eggs or egg whites and tofu. To most people's surprise the best source of protein may well be the humble bean. Beans are high-protein, low-fat and high-fibre, and they break down slowly in your digestive system, so you feel fuller longer. They can also be added to foods like soups and salads to boost their protein and fibre content. Nuts too are a fine source of protein, with a good monounsaturated fat content. However, because they are so high in fat, you must limit the quantity.

One of the most important things you should know about protein is to spread your daily allowance across all your meals. Too often we grab a hasty breakfast of coffee and toast—a protein-free meal. Lunch is sometimes not much better: a bowl of pasta with steamed vegetables or a green salad with garlic bread. Where's the protein? A typical afternoon snack of a cookie, piece of fruit or muffin contains not a gram of protein. Generally, it's not until dinner that we include protein in our meal, usually our entire daily recommended allowance plus some extra. Because protein is a critical brain food, providing amino acids for the neurotransmitters that relay messages in the brain, it would be better to load up on protein earlier in the day rather than later. That would give you an alert and active mind for your daily activities. However, as I have said, the best solution is to spread your protein consumption throughout the day. This will help keep you on the ball and feeling full.

Now that we know how carbohydrates, fats and proteins work in our digestive system and what makes us gain weight, let's use the science to put together an eating plan that will take off the extra pounds. First, though, let's look at how much weight you should be trying to lose.

TO SUM UP:
1. Include some protein in all your meals and snacks.
2. Eat only low-fat protein, preferably from both animal and vegetable sources.

Dear Rick,

Thank you so much for making a better life so easy to attain. I was 35 and 320 pounds with a family history of diabetes. I knew that I was destined to get the disease too unless I lost weight . . . I heard that a relative of mine who lives in Australia was following your diet. Once I read your book I knew it was the way to a new life . . . My wife and I have been on the G.I. Diet for five weeks and if I continue losing weight at this rate, by August I will be at my high school weight of 185 pounds and a normal BMI! My wife is also losing 5 pounds a week. That isn't as amazing as the complete change in the way I eat. I have cut out so much junk that I can't imagine ever going back to my old lifestyle. I feel so empowered. It took sixteen years to put the weight on, and it will take eight months to take it off. I'm undoing two years of neglect every month. Wow!

Your biggest fan,
Derek

CHAPTER TWO

How Much Weight Should I Lose?

In this age of excessively and often unhealthily skinny supermodels and TV stars, it's easy to lose sight of what is a healthy weight. Your skin, bones, organs, hair—everything—contribute to your total weight. The only part that you want to reduce is your excess fat, so that's what we have to determine.

There have been many techniques designed to measure excess fat, from measuring pinches of fat (which can be quite misleading) to convoluted formulas and tables requiring higher math. The traditional method, relating weight directly to height through the Metropolitan Life tables, does not tell you how much body fat you're carrying around your waist, hips and thighs, and that's the information you really need to know. So the best method is the Body Mass Index, or BMI. I've included a BMI table on pages 26 to 27 and it's very simple to use. Just find your height in the left vertical column and go across the table until you reach your weight. At the top of that column is your BMI, which is a pretty accurate estimate of the proportion of body fat you're carrying.

BMI values between 25 and 29 are classified as overweight, while those over 30 are classified as obese. If your BMI falls between 19 and 24, your weight is within the acceptable range. Because women generally have a smaller frame and lower muscle mass than men, they might want to target a BMI at the lower end of that range, while men should target a BMI at the higher end. If you are over 65 years, I suggest you allow yourself an extra 10 pounds to help protect you in case of a fall or long illness. Basically everyone has their own particular body makeup, metabolism and genes, so there are no hard and fast rules for exactly how much you should weigh. The BMI table is a guide, not an absolute.

Say you've decided to target a BMI of 22. Put your finger on the BMI number 22 and drop down until you reach your height, which is shown in the left margin. The number at that intersection is what your weight should be to achieve your BMI target. Let's look at an example: Mary is 5 feet 6 inches and weighs 180 pounds. Her current BMI is 29, but she'd like to have a BMI of 22. This means Mary has to lose 44 pounds in order to bring her to her 22 BMI goal of 136 pounds.

Another measurement that is important to know is your waist circumference. This measurement is an even better indication of your health than your weight is. Recent research has shown that abdominal fat acts almost like a separate organ in the body—only this "organ" is a destructive one. It releases harmful proteins and free fatty acids, increasing the risk of heart disease, stroke, cancer and diabetes. Thus women with a waist circumference of 35 inches or more and men with 37 inches or more are at risk of endangering their health. And women with a waist circumference of 37 inches or more and men with 40 inches or more are at serious risk of heart disease, stroke, cancer and diabetes. Doctors describe people with abdominal fat as apple-shaped.

To measure your waist, take a measuring tape and wrap it around your natural waist just above the navel. Don't be tempted to do a walk-down-the-beach-and-suck-it-in routine. Just stand in a relaxed position and keep the measuring tape from cutting into your flesh.

The 44 pounds that Mary has to lose are pounds of fat—Mary's energy storage tank. In order for her to lose weight she must access and draw down those fat cells. This reminds me of a peculiar contraption used in England during the Second World War. The famous double-decker buses had their upper deck converted into a natural gas tank, consisting of a large fabric balloon. When full, the balloon puffed up several feet above the top of the bus. As it proceeded along its route, the balloon slowly deflated, disappearing by the end of its destination, where it was re-inflated. That's how I visualize our body fat: a deflating balloon from which we draw down our energy, except that in our case the balloon is around our waist, hips and thighs!

BODY MASS

		NORMAL					OVERWEIGHT					OBESE	
BMI	**19**	**20**	**21**	**22**	**23**	**24**	**25**	**26**	**27**	**28**	**29**	**30**	**31**
HEIGHT						WEIGHT (POUNDS)							
4'10"	91	96	100	105	110	115	119	124	129	134	138	143	148
4'11"	94	99	104	109	114	119	124	128	133	138	143	148	153
5'0"	97	102	107	112	118	123	128	133	138	143	148	153	158
5'1"	100	106	111	116	122	127	132	137	143	148	153	158	164
5'2"	104	109	115	120	126	131	136	142	147	153	158	164	169
5'3"	107	113	118	124	130	135	141	146	152	158	163	169	175
5'4"	110	116	122	128	134	140	145	151	157	163	169	174	180
5'5"	114	120	126	132	138	144	150	156	162	168	174	180	186
5'6"	118	124	130	136	142	148	155	161	167	173	179	186	192
5'7"	121	127	134	140	146	153	159	166	172	178	185	191	198
5'8"	125	131	138	144	151	158	164	171	177	184	190	197	203
5'9"	128	135	142	149	155	162	169	176	182	189	196	203	209
5'10"	132	139	146	153	160	167	174	181	188	195	202	209	216
5'11"	136	143	150	157	165	172	179	186	193	200	208	215	222
6'0"	140	147	154	162	169	177	184	191	199	206	213	221	228
6'1"	144	151	159	166	174	182	189	197	204	212	219	227	235
6'2"	148	155	163	171	179	186	194	202	210	218	225	233	241
6'3"	152	160	168	176	184	192	200	208	216	224	232	240	248
6'4"	156	164	172	180	189	197	205	213	221	230	238	246	254

Source: U.S. National Heart, Lung and Blood Institute

INDEX (BMI)

	OBESE								EXTREME OBESITY					
	32	**33**	**34**	**35**	**36**	**37**	**38**	**39**	**40**	**41**	**42**	**43**	**44**	**45**
	WEIGHT (POUNDS)													
	153	158	162	167	172	177	181	186	191	196	201	205	210	215
	158	163	168	173	178	183	188	193	198	203	208	212	217	222
	163	168	174	179	184	189	194	199	204	209	215	220	225	230
	169	174	180	185	190	195	201	206	211	217	222	227	232	238
	175	180	186	191	196	202	207	213	218	224	229	235	240	246
	180	186	191	197	203	208	214	220	225	231	237	242	248	254
	186	192	197	204	209	215	221	227	232	238	244	250	256	262
	192	198	204	210	216	222	228	234	240	246	252	258	264	270
	198	204	210	216	223	229	235	241	247	253	260	266	272	278
	204	211	217	223	230	236	242	249	255	261	268	274	280	287
	210	216	223	230	236	243	249	256	262	269	276	282	289	295
	216	223	230	236	243	250	257	263	270	277	284	291	297	304
	222	229	236	243	250	257	264	271	278	285	292	299	306	313
	229	236	243	250	257	265	272	279	286	293	301	308	315	322
	235	242	250	258	265	272	279	287	294	302	309	316	324	331
	242	250	257	265	272	280	288	295	302	310	318	325	333	340
	249	256	264	272	280	287	295	303	311	319	326	334	342	350
	256	264	272	279	287	295	303	311	319	327	335	343	351	359
	263	271	279	287	295	304	312	320	328	336	344	353	361	369

So how do you draw down energy from your fat cells? By consuming fewer calories than your body needs. This will force your body to start using its fat stores to make up for the shortfall. Now, I know no one wants to hear about calories, particularly those of us who've tried long and hard to lose weight. Nevertheless, unless you are among those rare and blessed people whose metabolism and genetics enable them to eat as much as they want without gaining an ounce—and if you are, why would you be reading this book?—you, like me and the rest of us mere mortals, are doomed to the inevitable equation. But don't be disheartened: you can easily reduce your daily calorie intake without going hungry and without having to calculate the number of calories in everything you put in your mouth. All you have to do is eat low-G.I. foods (of course!) and adjust the ratio of carbohydrates, fats and proteins in your diet.

Ultimately, all food is a source of energy for our bodies, and we measure energy in calories. The average adult uses somewhere between 1,500 and 3,000 calories a day, depending upon level of activity, rate of metabolism and body weight. What people have been advised to do for decades is to get 55 percent of their calories from carbohydrates, 30 percent from fats and 15 percent from protein. But with our advancing knowledge of nutrition and how our digestive system works, this ratio is being challenged by many physicians and nutritionists. Accordingly, I recommend a modest adjustment to the traditional ratio. You should still get 55 percent of your calories from carbohydrates, but I am recommending that you eat less fat and a bit more protein than what has traditionally been advocated. A recent Harvard School of Public Health study involving over eighty thousand women concluded that a moderately high level of protein intake (24 percent) is beneficial to heart health. Also, the more one exercises, the more protein one needs. Athletes require up to twice the amount of protein as the average person. Though I certainly don't expect you to become an athlete, I will be encouraging more exercise in chapter 9.

SOURCE OF CALORIES—THE G.I. DIET

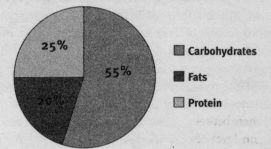

Okay, so we now have the ratio that will help us lose those extra pounds. It's all very fine in theory, but what does it mean in the real world? That's what the rest of this book is all about: how much of what to eat and when. I promised you a simple eating plan that reflects the real world we live in, and that is what I'll give you. The plan is divided into two phases. In Phase I you'll be reducing your caloric intake, burning off those excess fat cells and slimming down to a healthy, ideal weight. This phase takes between three and six months, and it's really a matter of simple math. A pound of fat contains around 3,600 calories. To lose that pound in one week you must reduce your caloric intake by around 500 calories per day (500 x 7 days = 3,500 calories). So if you want to lose twenty pounds, it will take twenty weeks. Here's an example: Mark weighs 180 pounds and he wants to lose 18 pounds. In order to lose a pound a week, Mark must reduce his calorie consumption by 3,500 calories per week. Based on this, it will take Mark 18 weeks to lose 18 pounds. But this formula is for people who have to lose about 10 percent of their body weight. If you have more to lose, the good news is that you will in all likelihood drop more pounds per week. The higher your BMI, the faster you will lose weight. People with a BMI of 30 and over frequently lose an average of 3 or more pounds per week.

If twenty weeks seems like a long time to be on a diet, think of it in terms of the rest of your life. What's half a year compared with the many, many years you'll spend afterwards with a slim, healthy body? This isn't a fad diet—fad diets don't work. The G.I. Diet is a wholesome and surefire route to permanent weight loss.

The reason I've included all this math is to help you understand this diet and how it's going to work for you. But I don't want you to think that you're going to have to do any calculations yourself! They're all built into the program. All you have to do is look at my food guide in the colour insert, which lists every food that you can think of in one of three categories based on the colours of the stoplight. Foods listed in the red-light or "stop" category are high-G.I, high-calorie foods. They include broad beans, melba toast and rice cakes, and they should be avoided. These foods are digested so quickly by your body that you soon become hungry again. Foods in the yellow-light or "caution" category, for example, muesli, corn and bananas, raise your insulin levels to the point where weight loss is less likely to happen, and should therefore be avoided in Phase I as well. The foods that will make you lose weight are the ones that are listed in the green-light or "go ahead" category. Fettuccine, basmati rice, grapes and many, many others are all green-light foods. Eat them and watch your weight drop.

When you've reached your target BMI, Phase II begins. Here, your calorie input and output are balanced. You're no longer trying to lose weight, so you can start eating foods from the yellow-light category from time to time. All you're doing at this point is maintaining your new weight. Sound simple? It is! So let's get going with Phase I.

TO SUM UP:

1. Set a realistic weight loss target. A BMI of 19 to 24 should be your goal.

2. In Phase I of the G.I. Diet you'll be reducing the number of calories you consume by adjusting your caloric intake ratio and by eating low-G.I., low-fat foods.

3. When you reach your target BMI, you'll start Phase II of the G.I. Diet, which evens out the number of calories you consume and expend.

Dear Rick,

Prior to reading your book, I was 177 pounds and was told by my doctor to read your book *The G.I. Diet*. I would like to let you know that I've since read it three times . . . Although my physician told me to lose 17 pounds, I have lost 25 pounds and am almost at a BMI of 22. This has been quite a learning process for me and I still can't believe that with proper nutrition and daily exercise this could happen. I have since had to alter all my clothes. (The seamstresses should thank you too!)

Thank you,

Jim

CHAPTER THREE

Phase I

Before we go any further, I'd like you to do a little assignment. Try to remember as best you can what you've been eating over the past seven days and fill in the "current" columns of the chart on the next page. This exercise will give you a bit of a reality check and help you to form a baseline or starting point from which you will build your new G.I. Diet program. Later in the book I will ask you to return to this page and record what you've been eating for the past week. I think you'll find the change very interesting—even enlightening.

DAY	BREAKFAST		LUNCH		DINNER		SNACKS	
	CURRENT	G.I. DIET	CURRENT	G.I. DIET	CURRENT	G.I. DIET	CURRENT	G.I. DIET
MONDAY								
TUESDAY								
WEDNESDAY								
THURSDAY								
FRIDAY								
SATURDAY								
SUNDAY								

With the theory and science of the G.I. Diet behind us, it's time to get practical! As you know, Phase I is the weight loss portion of the program, so we'll be sticking with low-G.I., low-fat foods, which we are categorizing as green light. In most cases you can eat as much of the green-light foods as you want. It's very important at this stage to eat frequently. This isn't a deprivation diet! So don't leave your digestive system with nothing to do. The saying "The devil finds work for idle hands" also applies to your stomach. If your digestive system is busy processing food and steadily supplying energy to your brain, you won't be looking for high-calorie snacks.

With that in mind, never skip breakfast. People who miss breakfast leave their stomachs empty from dinner to lunch the next day—often more than sixteen hours! No wonder they gorge themselves at lunch and then look for a sugar fix mid-afternoon as they run out of steam. Always eat three meals a day—breakfast, lunch and dinner—that contain approximately the same amount of energy (calories), as well as up to three snacks—one mid-morning, one mid-afternoon and one before bed. *Never use sugar*. Instead use a sugar substitute. And because liquids don't seem to trip our satiety mechanisms, don't waste your calorie allocation on beverages. Always drink water, skim milk and other no-cal or low-cal beverages.

So what can you eat? Let's talk about breakfast first. The following chart lists breakfast foods in the three colour-coded categories. For a comprehensive list, see the colour insert.

Breakfast

	RED	YELLOW	GREEN
PROTEIN			
Meat and Eggs	Regular bacon	Turkey bacon	Back bacon
	Sausages	Whole omega-3 eggs	Lean ham
	Whole regular eggs		Liquid eggs/ egg whites
Dairy	Cheese	Cream cheese (light)	Buttermilk
	Cottage cheese (whole or 2%)	Milk (1%)	Cheese (fat free)
	Cream	Sour cream (light)	Cottage cheese (1% or fat free)
	Milk (whole or 2%)	Yogurt (low fat with sugar)	Fruit yogurt (nonfat with sugar substitute)
	Sour cream		Milk (skim)
	Yogurt (whole or 2%)		Soy milk (plain, low fat)
CARBOHYDRATES			
Cereals	All cold cereals except those listed as yellow- or green-light	Kashi Go Lean Crunch	All-Bran
	Granola	Kashi Good Friends	Bran Buds
	Muesli (commercial)	Red River	Fibre First
		Shredded Wheat Bran	Homemade Muesli (see p. 87)
			Kashi Go Lean
			Oat bran
			Porridge (old-fashioned rolled oats)

	RED	YELLOW	GREEN
Breads/ Grains	Bagels	Crispbreads (with fibre)	100% stone-ground whole wheat*
	Baguette	Whole grain breads*	Crispbreads (high fibre, e.g., Wasa Fibre)*
	Cookies		Green-light muffins see pp. 172-75)
	Croissants		Homemade Granola Bars (see p. 176)
	Donuts		Whole-grain, high-fibre breads (2½–3 g fibre per slice)*
	Muffins		
	Pancakes/Waffles		
	White bread		
Fruits	Applesauce containing sugar	Apricots ** (fresh and dried)	Apples
	Canned fruit in syrup	Bananas	Berries
	Melons	Dried cranberries **	Cherries
	Most dried fruit	Fruit cocktail in juice	Grapefruit
		Kiwi	Grapes
		Mango	Oranges
		Papaya	Peaches
		Pineapple	Plums
Juices	Fruit drinks	Apple (unsweetened)	Eat the fruit rather than drink its juice
	Prune	Grapefruit (unsweetened)	
	Sweetened juices	Orange (unsweetened)	
	Watermelon	Pear (unsweetened)	

* Limit serving size (see page 63).

** For baking, it is okay to use a modest amount of dried apricots or cranberries.

	RED	YELLOW	GREEN
Vege-tables	French fries		Most vegetables
	Hash browns		

FATS			
	Butter	Most nuts	Almonds*
	Hard margarine	Natural nut butters	Canola oil*
	Peanut butter (regular and lite)	Natural peanut butter	Hazelnuts*
	Tropical oils	Soft margarine (non-hydrogenated)	Olive oil*
	Vegetable shortening	Vegetable oils	Soft margarine (nonhydrogenated, light)*

*Limit serving size (see page 63).

Juice

- Always eat the fruit or vegetable, rather than drink its juice. Juice is a processed product that is more rapidly digested than the parent fruit. To illustrate the point: diabetics who run into an insulin crisis and are in a state of hypoglycemia (low blood sugar) are usually given orange juice, which is the fastest way to get glucose into the bloodstream. A glass of juice has 2½ times the calories of a fresh whole orange.

Cereals

- Large-flake or slow-cooking porridge oats are the best choice for two reasons: oatmeal stays with you all morning, and it's great for your heart as it lowers cholesterol. (The cooking time is only around three minutes in the microwave.) Oat bran is also excellent.

- Among cold cereals, go for the high-fibre products—the ones that have at least 10 grams of fibre per serving. Fibre content is clearly indicated on cereal packages. Cereal manufacturers, to their credit, were among the first to voluntarily publish nutritional facts.

- High-fibre cereals are a great base to which fruit, nuts and yogurt may be added.

Dairy

- The beverage of choice is skim milk. I had a real problem with skim milk both on cereal and as a beverage, but I persevered. Move down from 2% to 1% to skim in stages. I find that 2% tastes like cream now!

- Yogurt is a real plus. But look for low- or no-fat versions with sugar substitute rather than sugar. Regular low-fat yogurts have nearly twice the calories as the versions with sweetener. (There has been a considerable amount of negative publicity, generated principally by the sugar industry, about sugar substitutes. This has triggered dozens of studies worldwide, none of which have shown any long-term risks to our health. These products are safe and of real value in calorie control. But, as with most foods, don't go overboard.)

- Cottage cheese is an excellent and filling source of protein. Again, go for the 1% or fat-free variety. Add fruit or light fruit spreads for flavour.

- Use other dairy products sparingly. Avoid most cheeses like the plague; their high saturated fat heads straight for your arteries. The dairy industry has a lot to answer for when it comes to our health. The success of their massive cheese advertising and promotion campaigns, often aimed at children, is reprehensible. If cheese is your thing, then go for the no-fat options or use stronger-flavoured ones, such as Stilton or feta, sprinkled sparingly as a flavour enhancer.

Bread

- Always use 100-percent stone-ground whole wheat, or any other whole-grain bread that has 2½ to 3 grams of fibre per slice. "Stone ground" is important because stones grind grain more coarsely than the steel rollers that grind most of our flour. The coarser the grind, the less the fibre is separated, resulting in a lower G.I.

Eggs

- Choose low-cholesterol, low-fat eggs in liquid form (250 ml carton = 5 eggs). Unlike regular eggs, which are high in cholesterol, eggs in liquid form are a great green-light product. Go for them.

Spreads

- Do not use butter. The latest premium brands of non-hydrogenated soft margarine are acceptable and the light versions even more so, but use sparingly.

- Avoid all fruit spreads where the first ingredient is sugar. Look for the "double fruit no added sugar" versions. These taste terrific and are remarkably low in calories. They are wonderful flavour boosters for oatmeal, high-fibre cereal and cottage cheese.

Bacon

- Sorry, but regular bacon is a red-light food. Acceptable alternatives are Canadian back bacon, turkey bacon and lean ham.

Coffee

- Coffee ideally should be decaffeinated (see page 66). Never add sugar and use only 1% or skim milk.

Lunch

Because lunch is the meal most of us eat outside the home, it can be the most problematic, limited by time, budget and availability considerations. There are, however, some practical guidelines. (For a complete list, see the colour insert.)

	RED	YELLOW	GREEN
PROTEIN			
Meat, Poultry, Fish and Eggs	Ground beef (more than 10% fat)	Ground beef (lean)	All fish and seafood, fresh or frozen (no batter or breading) or canned
	Hamburgers	Lamb (lean cuts)	Beef (lean cuts)
	Hot dogs	Pork (lean cuts)	Chicken/Turkey breast (skinless)
	Paté	Turkey bacon	Ground beef (extra-lean)
	Processed meats	Whole omega-3 eggs	Lean deli ham
	Regular bacon	Tofu	Liquid eggs (e.g., Break Free)
	Sausages		Tofu (low fat)
	Whole regular eggs		Veal
Dairy	Cheese	Milk (1%)	Cheese (fat free)
	Cottage cheese (whole or 2%)	Cheese (low fat)	Cottage cheese (1% or fat free)
	Cream cheese	Yogurt (low fat with sugar)	Fruit yogurt (nonfat with sugar substitute)
	Milk (whole or 2%)	Cream cheese (light)	Ice cream (low fat and no added sugar)
			Milk (skim)

	RED	YELLOW	GREEN
CARBOHYDRATES			
Breads/ Grains	Bagels	Crispbreads (with fibre, e.g., Ryvita High Fibre)	100% stone-ground whole wheat bread*
	Baguette/ Croissants	Pita (whole wheat)	Crispbreads (high fibre, e.g., Wasa Fibre
	Croutons	Tortillas (whole wheat)	Pasta* (fettuccine, spaghetti, penne, vermicelli, linguine, macaroni)
	Cake/Cookies	Whole grain breads*	Quinoa
	Hamburger/Hotdog Buns		Rice (basmati, wild, brown, long grain)
	Macaroni and cheese		Whole-grain, high-fibre breads (2½–3 g fibre per slice)*
	Muffins/Donuts		
	Noodles (canned or instant)		
	Pancakes/Waffles		
	Pasta filled with cheese or meat		
	Pizza		
	Rice (short grain, white, instant)		

	RED	YELLOW	GREEN	
Fruits/ Vegetables	Broad beans	Apricots	Apples	Lettuce
	French fries	Artichokes	Arugula	Mushrooms
	Melons	Bananas	Asparagus	Olives*
	Most dried fruit	Beets	Avocado*	Onions
	Parsnips	Corn	Beans (green/wax)	Oranges (all varieties)

* Limit serving size (see page 63).

RED	YELLOW	GREEN	
Potatoes (mashed or baked)	Kiwi	Bell peppers	Peaches
Rutabaga	Mangoes	Blackberries	Pears
	Papaya	Broccoli	Peas
	Pineapple	Brussels sprouts	Peppers (hot)
	Potatoes (boiled)	Cabbage	Pickles
	Squash	Carrots	Plums
	Sweet Potatoes	Cauliflower	Potatoes boiled new)*
	Yams	Celery	Radishes
		Cherries	Raspberries
		Cucumbers	Snow peas
		Eggplant	Spinach
		Grapefruit	Strawberries
		Grapes	Tomatoes
		Leeks	Zucchini
		Lemons	
RED	YELLOW	GREEN	

FATS

RED	YELLOW	GREEN
Butter	Mayonnaise (light)	Almonds*
Hard margarine	Most nuts	Canola oil*
Mayonnaise	Natural peanut butter (no added sugar)	Mayonnaise (fat free)
Peanut butter (regular, lite)	Salad dressings (light)	Olive oil*
Salad dressings (regular)	Soft margarine (nonhydrogenated)	Salad dressings (low fat, low sugar)
Tropical oils		Soft margarine (non-hydrogenated, light)

* Limit serving size (see page 63).

RED	YELLOW	GREEN
Soups		
All cream-based soups	Canned chicken noodle	Chunky bean and vegetable soups
Canned black bean	Canned lentil	(e.g., Campbell's
Canned green pea	Canned tomato	Healthy Request,
Canned puréed vegetable		Healthy Choice and Too Good To Be True)
Canned split pea		

Sandwiches

- Sandwiches are probably the most popular choice for lunch in North America, and they usually have a high G.I. and are high in calories. But you don't have to cut sandwiches out of your diet. To lower their impact on your hips, choose sandwiches made with whole wheat or whole grain bread, the grittier the better. Then take off the top layer of the bread and eat the sandwich open-faced. Watch out for mayonnaise—it's often hidden in egg, chicken and tuna salad. Always ask for no mayo—unless it's non- or low fat. Also request no butter or margarine on bread. Hummus or mustard are good alternatives.

Salads

- Though usually green light, salads are often short on protein. Add beans, salmon, tofu, chicken or turkey breast. Use only low-fat dressings that are also low in sugar. For some green-light salad suggestions, see pages 92 to 95 and 128 to 135.

Pasta

- Though most pastas range in the moderate G.I. category, some are clearly preferable to others. A rule of thumb is that thicker pastas are better. Pasta is a villain in our obesity problem not because of any issue with pasta itself—a moderate-G.I. and low-fat (although high-calorie) product—but due to the quantities we eat. Italians are aghast at the huge bowls of pasta we consume as our main course. They quite correctly view pasta as an appetizer or a side dish. We typically view it as the bulk of the meal, with sauce and a few pieces of protein on top.

  Because it's difficult when dining out to order a partial plate of pasta, it's best to avoid it completely. If you are able to obtain a side order, then limit the quantity to cover a quarter of the plate (about ¼ cup) and ask for low-fat sauce options. Please, no alfredo. Whole grain pasta is your best choice.

Soups

- A chunky bean or vegetable soup followed by fish or chicken makes an ideal lunch. Beware of cream-based or puréed vegetable soups; they are high in fat and heavily processed, therefore red light all the way.

Potatoes

- Since it's almost impossible to get plain, boiled new potatoes when eating out (see page 56), always ask your server for double vegetables in lieu of potatoes. In two years, after dozens of requests, I've never been refused.

Rice
- Eat basmati, brown, wild or long-grain rice only, and in quantities to cover no more than a quarter of your plate. Avoid rice if it's glutinous and sticky.

Dessert
- Nonfat yogurt sweetened with a sugar substitute is a terrific choice. Always eat some fruit. I keep a supply of apples, pears, peaches and grapes, depending on the season, in my office. Stay away from most other desserts.

Fast Food
- The simple answer to "Should I visit fast-food outlets for lunch?" is NO. With a few exceptions, fast food is loaded with saturated fat and calories, with rarely a gram of fibre in sight. For example, a Quarter Pounder with cheese hits you with just under 500 calories and over half your day's quota of fat. Even the carrot muffin comes loaded with calories and fat. Merely being in the presence of all those tempting burgers, fries and shakes makes your challenges more difficult—so stay away if at all possible. I can assure you that after a few months on the G.I. Diet, even the idea of fast food will turn you off. With your face pressed to the window of McDonald's, you'll watch with amazement what the heavyweights are putting away—straight to their waists and hips. That could have been you!

  If your alternatives are limited, here is how you can sucessfully navigate through this gastronomic minefield.

Salads: The introduction of salads at fast food chains such as McDonald's has been the one bright light in the industry. They make good choices providing you do not use the whole packet of dressing, which can double the calorie content of the meal. Go for the low-fat dressing options and use only half the packet. Steer clear of Caesar salads.

Submarines: Subway is to be congratulated as the pace-setter in the fast food industry. They have a wide range of low-fat subs to choose from. Ask for a whole wheat roll and avoid the cheese and mayo unless they're low-fat. Then eat the sandwich open-faced. A word of caution: avoid Subway's low-carb Atkins wraps; they're loaded with fat and calories.

Burgers: Dispose of the top of the bun and don't order cheese or bacon. Keep it as simple as possible.

Fries: DON'T. A medium order of McDonald's fries contains 17 grams of fat (mostly saturated), about 50 percent of your total daily allowance.

Milkshakes: DON'T. The saturated fat and calorie levels are unbelievable.

Wraps: An increasingly popular alternative to the traditional sandwich is a wrap. Ask for a whole wheat tortilla and pass on the cheese.

Pizza: Pizza is red light due to both its high-G.I. crust and the massive amount of saturated (bad) fat from the traditional cheese-based toppings. If you are fortunate enough to have a restaurant that will make you a custom pizza, then ask for a super-thin whole wheat crust, tomato sauce, lots of vegetables, fresh herbs and some sliced chicken breast (and *no* cheese). You can also make this at home using a split whole wheat pita bread (half thickness) as the crust.

Fish: An excellent choice providing there's no batter or breaded coating.

Chinese: The two things to watch for are the rice and the sauces, especially the sweet ones, which are high in sugar. Rice is usually a problem, as most restaurants use a glutinous high-G.I. rice whose grains tend to stick together. If you can be assured the rice is either basmati or long grain and doesn't clump together, then okay, but limit the quantity to a quarter of your plate.

Mexican: Along with unacceptably high levels of fat, especially saturated, most Mexican fast food also has extremely high sodium (salt) levels. Many meals contain enough salt for over half your total daily requirement! Excessive levels of salt boost blood pressure, which can in turn lead to heart attacks and stroke.

Snacks

Because it's a bad idea to leave your stomach empty, snacks are an important part of the G.I. Diet. But I'm afraid you'll have to avoid the customary choices like muffins, cookies and chips, all high-G.I. foods that are calorie-dense. Two hours after eating them you've added a few more fat cells and are feeling hungry again. These foods are just not worth the trouble.

Phase I snacks include fruit, nonfat yogurt sweetened with sugar substitute, 1% cottage cheese and raw vegetables. You might also want to explore the world of food bars. Stay away from the expensive high-carbohydrate, high-calorie sugar bars, choosing instead those that have a more balanced ratio of carbohydrates, fats and proteins. Half a Balance Bar or Zone Bar is an excellent snack, and so are most bars that weigh between 50 and 65 grams and have around 200 calories. They should contain 20 to 30 grams of carbohydrates, 12 to 15 grams of protein and only 5 grams of fat. Check labels carefully.

If you bake your own low-G.I. muffins and granola bars (the recipes are in chapter 8), they also make good snacks. You can freeze a batch or two and reheat them in the microwave.

SNACKS	RED	YELLOW	GREEN
	Bagels	Bananas	Almonds**
	Candy	Dark chocolate (70% cocoa)	Applesauce (unsweetened)
	Cookies	Ice cream (low fat)	Canned peaches/pears in juice or water
	Crackers	Most nuts**	Cottage cheese (1% or fat free)
	Donuts	Popcorn (air popped)	Extra low-fat cheese (e.g., Laughing Cow Light, Boursin Light)
	Flavoured gelatin (all varieties)		Fruit yogurt (nonfat with sugar substitute)
	French fries		Food bars*
	Ice cream		Green-light muffins (see pp. 172–74)
	Muffins (commercial)		Hazelnuts**
	Popcorn (regular)		Homemade cookies (see pp.180–85)
	Potato chips		Homemade Granola Bars (see p. 176)
	Pretzels		Ice cream (low fat and
	Pudding		no added sugar, e.g.,
	Raisins		Breyers Premium Fat
	Rice cakes		Free, Nestlé's Legend
	Sorbet		No Added Sugar)
	Tortilla chips		Most fresh fruit
	Trail mix		Most fresh vegetables
	White bread		Pickles
			Pumpkin seeds
			Sugar-free hard candies
			Sunflower seeds

* 180–225 calorie bars, e.g. Zone or Balance Bars; ½ bar per serving

** Limit serving size (see page 63).

Dinner

Dinner, traditionally, is the main meal of the day—and the one where most of us blow our diet to shreds. Unlike breakfast and lunch, dinner doesn't usually have any time or availability constraints (although juggling our schedules along with our children's can sometimes make this a moot point).

The typical North American dinner comprises three things: meat or fish; potato, pasta or rice; and vegetables. Together, these foods provide an assortment of carbohydrates, proteins and fats, along with other minerals and vitamins essential to our health.

(For a complete list, see the colour insert).

	RED	YELLOW	GREEN
PROTEIN			
Meat, Poultry, Fish and Eggs	Breaded fish and seafood	Ground beef (lean)	All fish and seafood (not breaded or canned in oil)
	Fish canned in oil		
	Ground beef (more than 10% fat)	Lamb (lean cuts)	Beef (lean cuts)
	Hamburgers	Pork (lean cuts)	Chicken breast (skinless)
	Hot dogs	Whole omega-3 eggs	Ground beef (extra lean)
	Processed meats		Lean deli ham
	Sausages		Low-cholesterol liquid eggs
	Sushi		Turkey breast (skinless)
	Whole regular eggs		Veal
Dairy	Cheese	Cheese (low fat)	Cheese (fat free)

	RED	YELLOW	GREEN
	Cottage cheese (whole or 2%)	Milk (1%)	Cottage cheese (1% or fat free)
	Milk (whole or 2%)	Sour cream (light)	Fruit yogurt (nonfat with sugar substitute)
	Sour cream	Yogurt (low fat)	Milk (skim)
	Yogurt (whole or 2%)		Soy milk (plain, low fat)

CARBOHYDRATES

Breads/ Grains	RED	YELLOW	GREEN
	Bagels	Pita (whole wheat)	100% stone-ground whole wheat*
	Baguette/Croissants	Whole grain breads*	Pasta* (fettuccine, spaghetti, penne,
	Cake/Cookies		vermicelli, linguine,
	Macaroni & cheese		macaroni)
	Muffins/Donuts		
	Noodles (canned or instant)		Quinoa
	Pasta filled with cheese or meat		Rice* (basmati, wild, brown, long grain)
	Pizza		Whole-grain, high-fibre breads (2½–3 g fibre per slice)
	Rice (short grain white, instant)		
	Tortillas		

Fruits/ Vegeta-bles	RED	YELLOW	GREEN	
	Broad beans	Apricots	Apples	Lettuce
	French fries	Bananas	Asparagus	Mushrooms
	Melons	Beets	Arugula	Olives*
	Most dried fruit	Corn	Beans (green/wax)	Onions

* Limit serving size (see page 63)

RED	YELLOW		GREEN	
Potatoes (mashed or baked)	Kiwi	Bell peppers	Oranges (all varieties)	
	Mangoes	Blackberries	Peaches	
	Papaya	Broccoli	Pears	
	Pineapple	Brussels sprouts	Peas	
	Pomegranates	Cabbage	Peppers (hot)	
	Potatoes (boiled)	Carrots	Pickles	
	Squash	Cauliflower	Plums	
	Sweet Potatoes	Celery	Potatoes (boiled new)	
	Yams	Cherries	Radishes	
		Cucumbers	Raspberries	
		Eggplant	Snow peas	
		Grapefruit	Spinach	
		Grapes	Strawberries	
		Leeks	Tomatoes	
		Lemons	Zucchini	
RED	YELLOW		GREEN	

Fats

RED	YELLOW	GREEN
Butter	Corn oil	Almonds*
Hard margarine	Mayonnaise (light)	Canola oil*
Mayonnaise	Most nuts	Hazelnuts*
Peanut butter (regular, lite)	Salad dressings (light)	Mayonnaise (fat free)
Salad dressings (regular)	Soft margarine (nonhydrogenated)	Olive oil*
Tropical oils	Vegetable oils	Pistachios*

* Limit serving size (see page 63)

	RED	YELLOW	GREEN
	Vegetable Shortening	Walnuts	Salad dressings (low fat, low sugar)
			Soft margarine (non-hydrogenated, light)

Soups

	RED	YELLOW	GREEN
	All cream-based soups	Canned chicken noodle	Chunky bean and vegetable soups
	Canned black bean	Canned lentil	(e.g., Campbell's
	Canned green pea	Canned tomato	Healthy Request,
	Canned puréed vegetable		Healthy Choice and Too Good To Be True)
	Canned split pea		Homemade soups with green-light ingredients

Meat/Fish

- Most meats contain saturated (bad) fat, so it's important to buy lean cuts or trim off all the visible fat. A loin steak trimmed to only a quarter-inch of fat can have up to twice the fat of a steak with no trim. Obviously, some cuts of meat intrinsically have a higher fat content. Check the Meat/Fish section in the colour insert.

- Chicken and turkey breasts are excellent choices *provided all the skin is removed.*

- Fish and seafood are also excellent choices unless they've been breaded. Though certain fish, such as salmon, have a relatively high oil content, this oil is extremely beneficial to your health, especially heart health.

- In terms of quantity, the best measure for meat or fish is your palm. The portion should be about the size of the palm of your hand and about as thick. Another good visual is a pack of cards—so my friends with small palms tell me!

Potatoes

- The G.I. rating of potatoes ranges from moderate to high, depending on the type and how they are cooked and served. In the lowest G.I. category are boiled new potatoes served whole or sliced, two to three per serving. (The G.I. for boiled new potatoes is 56, while baked have a G.I. of 84.) All other versions are strictly red light.

Pasta

- As mentioned earlier, the serving size is critical. Pasta should be a side dish and not form the base of the meal. In other words, it should take up only a quarter of your plate. Whole wheat pasta, available at most natural food stores and increasingly in your local supermarket, is preferable. Allow 35 grams of dried pasta, or ¾ cup cooked, per serving.

Rice

- Rice has a broad G.I. range. The best choices are basmati, wild, brown or long-grain. These rices contain a starch, amylose, that breaks down more slowly than other rices. Again, serving size is critical. Allow three tablespoons of dry rice per serving, or ⅔ cup cooked.

Vegetables/Salad

- This is where you can go wild. Eat as many vegetables and as much salad as you like. In fact, this should be the backbone of your meal. Virtually all vegetables are ideal. Try to have a side salad with your daily dinner.

- Watch out for salad dressings. Use only low-fat and fat-free ones, and check sugar content as manufacturers often bump up the sugar as they reduce the fat.

- Serve two or three varieties of vegetables for dinner. Frozen bags of mixed, unseasoned vegetables are inexpensive and convenient.

Desserts

- This is one of the most troublesome issues in any weight control program. Desserts usually taste great, but they tend to be loaded with sugar and fat—a real guilt-inducing situation! As the last course in most meals, desserts often fall into the "Should I or shouldn't I?" category.

  The good news is that dessert should be a part of your meal. There are a broad range of low-G.I., low-calorie alternatives that taste great and are good for you. Virtually any fruit qualifies (though hold off on the bananas and raisins) and there are numerous low-fat, low-sugar dairy products such as yogurt and ice cream. You won't be eating apple pie à la mode, but you could be enjoying applesauce with yogurt, or even a meringue with fresh or frozen berries.

Portions

Understanding portions is essential if the G.I. Diet is to work for you. Since most vegetables and fruits have a low G.I. rating and are low in calories and fat, they are the most important food group in the G.I. Diet. However, both the Canadian and U.S. governments suggest that grains should be the most important food group. If you look at the United States Department of Agriculture's Food Pyramid on the next page, you will see that it suggests grains should be the largest component of your diet, followed by vegetables and fruit. But by giving grains priority, governments and most nutritionists are promoting the leading cause of overweight and obesity. The Mayo Clinic has recently changed its Healthy Weight Pyramid to promote vegetables and fruits as the base of a healthy diet, rather than grains, and this is exactly what the G.I. Diet recommends. (See the G.I. Diet Food Pyramid on page 60.)

Dear Rick,

I just wanted to say that the day I read your article in *Woman's World* was the day my life changed. I have been on the G.I. Diet for ten weeks and have lost 40 pounds! I absolutely love this plan and find it so easy to live with. My husband and I can still go out to eat and not feel deprived of food or fun!! Thank you for all you have done for me.

Merrill

USDA FOOD PYRAMID

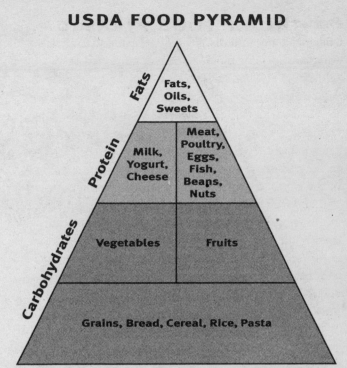

Source: U.S. Department of Agriculture

THE G.I. FOOD PYRAMID

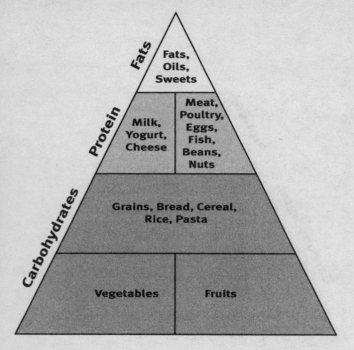

To translate the pyramid to your dinner plate, dish out enough vegetables to cover 50 percent of your plate, enough meat, poultry or fish to cover 25 percent of your plate, and enough rice, pasta or potatoes to cover the remaining 25 percent. Don't bend the rules by piling your food too high!

Below is a diagram of the way we traditionally visualize our dinner plate followed by the healthier G.I. Diet version.

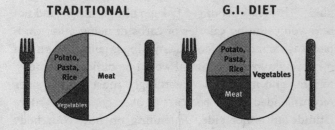

TRADITIONAL

Potato,
Pasta,
Rice   Meat

Vegetables

G.I. DIET

Potato,
Pasta,
Rice   Vegetables

Meat

Serving Size

Some nutritionists contend that today's weight issues are as much to do with serving size as with the type of food we eat. There is a great deal of truth to this. The "Big Mac" mentality has permeated our thinking. If one serving tastes terrific, think what two can do!

A trip to the movies encapsulates the problem. All popcorn, drinks and candy come in giant sizes only. The fast-food industry in particular has recognized our desire to treat ourselves when we eat out by ordering larger servings, and they do everything to encourage that tendency. Food is a relatively cheap commodity, especially when it is high in low-cost simple carbohydrates such as sugar and flour. That is why fast-food companies can offer bigger servings at very little incremental cost.

As in most things, common sense should be your guide. This book promised to keep things simple and not have you counting calories or carbs or using other complex ways to measure food. If anything is going to turn you off a weight-loss program, it would be difficult formulas, weights and measures. Accordingly, most serving sizes recommended in this book are an average. There is some latitude on either side, depending on how your body weight varies from the broad average—125 to 150 pounds for women and 140 to 175 for men. Adjust serving sizes down if you fall below the average, up if you are over. But to make it work and keep things simple, you have to do your part by using your own judgment. As with juries and democracy, the common sense of the public should not be underestimated!

While you can generally eat as much of the green-light foods as you like, there are a few exceptions which are listed on the next page.

Green-Light Serving Sizes

Avocado	¼ of the fruit
Crispbreads (with high fibre, e.g., Wasa Fibre)	2 crispbreads
Green-light breads (which have at least 2½ to 3 grams of fibre per slice)	1 slice
Green-light cereals	½ cup
Green-light nuts	8 to 10
Margarine (nonhydrogenated, light)	2 teaspoons
Meat, fish, poultry	4 ounces (about the size of a pack of cards)
Olive/canola oil	1 teaspoon
Olives	4 to 5
Pasta	¾ cup cooked
Potatoes (boiled new)	2 to 3
Rice (basmati, brown, long grain)	⅔ cup cooked
PHASE II	
Chocolate (70% cocoa)	2 squares
Red wine	1 5-ounce glass

The Family

One of the most frequent questions I am asked is whether the G.I. Diet is suitable for all members of the family, including children—and indeed it is. Phase II is a healthy way to eat for everyone, even if they don't need to lose any weight. Phase I is recommended for anyone who needs to reduce. If you think your child may be overweight, it is critical that you get your doctor's confirmation. Kids often put on weight prior to a growth spurt, and it's not something you should necessarily worry about. However childhood obesity in this country has tripled over the past twenty-five years, so it's important to introduce children to good eating habits. Children should always eat a nutritious breakfast (not sugary cereals), lunch, dinner and snacks made up of green- and yellow-light foods. Fresh fruit, vegetables, chicken, fish, yogurt, whole wheat bread, pasta, porridge and nuts are all kid-friendly foods that will see to their nutritional needs. Remember that growing children need sufficient fat in their diet—the good kind found in nuts, fish and vegetable oils.

If your doctor agrees that your child is overweight, gently introduce him or her to the Phase I way of eating. Don't put pressure on children to lose weight, simply encourage healthy food choices. And allow them to enjoy special treats on holidays and occasions such as birthdays and Halloween.

Vegetarians

I was surprised at the number of vegetarians who wrote me asking whether the G.I. Diet was right for them. Most vegetarians I know don't need to lose weight. But if you do, the G.I. Diet is certainly the program for you. Just continue to substitute vegetable protein for animal protein—something you've been doing all along. However, because most vegetable protein sources, such as beans, are encased in fibre, your digestive system may not be getting the maximum protein benefit. So try to add easily digestible protein boosters like tofu and soy protein powder.

You will find several vegetarian recipes in chapter 8, as well as suggestions on how to convert some recipes with meat to meatless.

Beverages

Since 70 percent of our body is made up of water, it's hardly surprising that drinking fluids is an important part of any dietary program. Most dieticians recommend eight glasses of fluid per day. This sounds a bit steep to me, and every time I make a conscious effort to comply I find myself running for the bathroom every couple of hours!

If you set out to drink eight glasses, in reality you end up consuming a great deal more than that. The reason is that we take in a great deal of fluid without being conscious of it. Add together other liquids you consume such as milk in cereal, and soft drinks, along with the water that makes up a great deal of the bulk of most fruits and vegetables, and you easily end up taking in several cups a day without even trying. *So the rule of thumb is: drink at least a glass of water with each of your three main meals and with each snack.*

Now, what to drink?

Water

The cheapest and best choice is plain, simple water. Try to drink an 8-ounce glass of water *before* each meal and snack, for two reasons. First, having your stomach partly filled with liquid before the meal means you will feel full more quickly, thus reducing the temptation to overeat. Second, you won't be tempted to "wash down" your food before it's been sufficiently chewed, thus upsetting your digestive system.

Soft Drinks

If water is too boring for you, go for sugar-free soft drinks, preferably also caffeine-free (see Coffee, below). Remember, the sugar in a drink is less satisfying than an equal quantity of sugar in food, so don't waste your calorie intake quota.

Skim Milk

My personal preference of beverage is skim milk, at least with breakfast and lunch. It's an ideal green-light food, and since most lunches tend to be protein deficient, drinking skim milk is a good way of making up some of the shortfall.

Coffee

The principal problem with coffee is caffeine. Caffeine stimulates insulin production, which encourages appetite. So try to curb your caffeine intake by limiting yourself to a cup of coffee per day. An alternative is decaffeinated coffee—no hardship given the delicious range of decaffeinated options available today.

As an experiment I asked a group of dinner guests whether they preferred caffeinated or decaffeinated coffee. It split about fifty-fifty. I then served decaffeinated coffee (a plug for Starbucks here) to everyone and asked how they liked it. I received more applause from those who had asked for caffeinated than from the dedicated decaf aficionados! I rest my case.

Tea

Tea has considerably less caffeine than coffee. Both black and green teas also contain an antioxidant property that appears to carry a significant heart health benefit. In fact there are higher quantities of flavonoids (antioxidants) in tea than in any vegetable tested. Two cups of tea have the same amount of antioxidants as seven cups of orange juice or twenty of apple juice. Maybe my ninety-three-year-old mother and her tea-drinking cronies are on to something.

So, tea in moderation is fine. If you are looking for alternative teas that are completely caffeine-free, there has been an explosion of flavoured herbal and fruit options, though they don't have the antioxidant characteristics of real tea. In fact, as I'm writing this, I'm drinking English Toffee tea—delicious! These teas are a lot of fun and taste great.

Fruit Drinks/Juices

Fruit drinks contain a large amount of sugar, are calorie-dense and definitely belong on the red-light list.

Fruit juices are preferable, but as we discussed earlier, it is always better to eat the fruit or vegetable rather than drink its juice. Remember, the more work your body has to do to break down food, the better. There is nothing worse than an idle stomach!

Alcohol

I'm sure this is the section that most readers fast-forwarded to. Well, it's a good news, bad news story.

The good news is that alcohol in moderation (and we'll discuss moderation in chapter 7) is not only acceptable but, as you'll learn later, can even be good for your health.

The bad news is that alcohol in general is a disaster for weight control. Alcohol is easily metabolized by the body, which means increased insulin production, a drop in blood sugar levels, and demand from the body for more alcohol or food to boost those sagging sugar levels. This is a vicious circle that can play havoc with your weight loss plans. To make things worse, most alcoholic drinks are loaded with empty calories.

So, NO ALCOHOL at all in Phase I.

TO SUM UP:
1. In Phase I eat exclusively green-light foods, i.e., those with a low glycemic, saturated fat, and calorie rating.
2. Eat three principal meals of equal nutritional value per day plus three between-meal snacks.
3. Drink lots of water or diet soft drinks, including an 8-ounce glass before or with each meal and snack. And don't touch caffeine or alcohol until Phase II!
4. Moderation and common sense are your guides for determining serving portions.

Dear Rick,

I decided to give the G.I. Diet a try . . . The first few days were rough—caffeine withdrawal headaches are not pretty. But I stuck to it, and after the sugars were gone from my body, I noticed that the cravings diminished dramatically. I can honestly say that this is the easiest, most logical food plan I've ever followed. This body that used to crave cookies and doughnuts now gets its sugar fix from an orange or a glass of caffeine-free, sugar-free soda . . . As of yesterday, I have lost 19 pounds. I feel great, and for the first time in a long time, have the confidence that I can do this!!!

Vicki

Ready, Set, Go!

Ready

By now, I hope you understand the principles of the G.I.
Diet and are totally convinced that the plan is going to
work for you for the rest of your life. All that's left is to take
the plunge. This is what I call the READY stage, and it is
perhaps the most agonizing part of the journey.

The best advice I can give comes from my own experience. I knew I had to lose twenty pounds to take me to the
22 BMI target weight. On the advice of a friend I gathered
together a number of books (diet books!) and piled them on
my bathroom scale until they totalled twenty pounds. I
then put them in a backpack and carried them around the
house one Sunday morning. By noon the weight was really
bugging me. What a relief it was to take the bag off my
back! So the question was, did I want to carry that excess
twenty pounds of fat around with me each and every day, or

lose it and gain the sense of lightness and freedom I experienced after the backpack came off?

I urge you to try the same exercise. Identify how much weight you want to lose by using the BMI chart on pages 26 to 27. Bundle up a sufficient number of books to equal that weight and carry them on your back or shoulder, or around your waist, for a few hours. Remember, that's the excess weight you are permanently carrying around with you. No wonder you feel exhausted! And that's one of the principal benefits of the G.I. Diet: not only will you look and feel great, but you will rediscover all that energy and zip you had in your teens and twenties, which you thought had been lost forever.

SET

Wondering what to do first? Well, let me suggest that you proceed in the following manner:

1. Baseline

Before you do anything else, get your vital statistics on record. Measuring progress is a great motivator. You will find a detachable log sheet on page 239 to keep in the bathroom and record your weekly progress. There are two key measurements. The first is weight. Always weigh yourself at the same time of day, because a meal or bowel movement can throw out your weight by a couple of pounds. First thing in the morning, before you eat breakfast, is a good time. The other important measurement is your waist. Measure at your natural waistline—usually just above the navel while standing in a relaxed, normal posture. The tape should be snug but not indenting the skin.

Record both measurements on the bathroom log. I've added a Comments column to the log sheet where you can note how you're feeling, or any unusual events in the past week that might have some bearing on your progress.

2. Pantry

Clear out your pantry, fridge and freezer of all red- and yellow-light products. Give them to a food bank or to your neighbours. If the products aren't around, you won't be tempted to eat or drink them.

3. Shopping

Stock up at home on products that get a green light. You will find a detachable shopping list on pages 228 and 229 to take with you to the grocery store. There are a few yellow-light products that have been asterisked, and these can be used sparingly during your Phase I weight loss period. After a couple of shopping trips, selecting the right products will become second nature.

Although we've tried to provide a broad range of products, we could not hope to cover all the thousands of brands available in most supermarkets. This means you have to check labels when in doubt. Look for four key numbers:

1. Serving size: Is this realistic? Often manufacturers who are concerned about the fat, cholesterol or calories of that product will identify a serving size smaller than is realistic. You'll see this on the labels of many high-sugar cereals.

2. Calories: Remember that this number is based on the serving size, which should be realistic.

3. Fat: Look for a minimum ratio of 3 grams of poly- or monounsaturated fat to each gram of saturated fat. Keep total fat to less than 10 grams per serving.

4. Fibre: Since fibrous foods have a lower G.I., look for a minimum of 4 to 5 grams of fibre per serving.

Basically, shop for foods that are low-calorie, low-fat (especially saturated) and high-fibre. That's the formula for all our green-light products: they have a low G.I., are low in saturated fat and are calorie-light. By eating these foods you will reduce your calorie intake without going hungry.

You will be buying considerably more fruit and vegetables than previously, so be a little daring and try some varieties that are new to you. There's a wonderful world of fresh and frozen produce just waiting for you to enjoy!

Caution: Don't go food shopping with an empty stomach or you'll end up buying items that don't belong on the G.I. Diet!

GO

Now that the difficult part is done, it's plain sailing from here. Don't be surprised if you lose more than one pound per week in the first few weeks, as your body adjusts to the new regimen. Most of that weight will be water, not fat. Remember, 70 percent of our body weight is water.

Don't worry if from time to time you "fall off the wagon," eating or drinking with friends and going outside the program. That's the real world, and though it will marginally delay your target date, it's more important that you not feel as though you're living in a straitjacket. I probably live about 90 percent within the program and 10 percent outside—by choice. The fact is, I feel better and more energized when on the program and rarely feel deprived. However, in Phase I, try to keep these lapses to a minimum; you will be able to allow yourself more leeway once you have achieved your target weight.

If you want further proof or reassurance that your new way of eating is really working, try this test. After eight weeks on the G.I. Diet, break all the rules and have a lunch consisting of a whole pizza with the works, a bread roll and a beer or regular soft drink. While you're at it, finish up with a slice of pie. I'll spare you the ice cream.

I did just that, and by about three in the afternoon I could hardly keep awake. I felt listless and worn out. I hadn't planned on eating so much but got caught up in a fellow employee's farewell lunch. The reason for my afternoon fatigue (which you've likely figured out for yourself) was the combination of high-G.I. foods (pizza, bread roll, beer and pie), which led to a rapid spike in my blood sugar level. The resulting rush of insulin drained this sugar from my blood and caused my sugar levels to drop precipitously, leaving my brain and muscles starved of energy, i.e., in a hypoglycemic state. No wonder I couldn't keep my eyes open.

Here are some tips to keep you motivated, especially when your resolve starts flagging (as it inevitably will from time to time):

1. Maintain a weekly progress log. (A removable log sheet appears on page 239.) Nothing is more motivating than success.

2. Set up a reward system. Buy yourself a small gift when you achieve a predetermined weight goal—perhaps a gift for every three pounds lost.

3. Identify family members or friends who will be your cheerleaders. Make them active participants in your plan. Even better, find a friend who will join the plan for mutual support.

4. Avoid acquaintances and haunts that may encourage your old behaviours. You know who I mean!

5. Try adding what my friend calls a special "spa" day to your week—a day when you are *especially good* with your program. This gives you some extra credit in your weight loss account to draw on when the inevitable relapse occurs.

6. Sign up for the free G.I. Diet newsletter to learn from readers' experiences and keep up-to-date on the latest developments in diet and health. Details at **www. gidiet.com**.

TO SUM UP:

1. Try the weighted backpack test.
2. Take baseline weight and waist measurements.
3. Clear the pantry, fridge and freezer of all red- and yellow-light products.
4. Shop for green-light products to restock your pantry, fridge and freezer.
5. Follow the six tips above this box, and do keep a record of your progress.
6. *Go for it!*

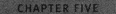

CHAPTER FIVE

The Green-Light Glossary

The following is a summary of the most popular green-light foods. For a full green-light list, see the colour insert.

Almonds	This is the perfect nut in that it has the highest monounsaturated fat (good fat) content of any nut, and recent research indicates that almonds can significantly lower LDL, or bad, cholesterol. They are also excellent sources of Vitamin E, fibre and protein. They provide a great boost to the beneficial fat content of your meals, especially at breakfast or in salads and desserts. Because all nuts are high in calories, use them in moderation.
Apples	A real staple. Use fresh as a snack or dessert. Unsweetened applesauce is ideal with cereals, or with cottage cheese as a snack.
Barley	An excellent supplement to soups.
Beans (legumes)	If there's one food you can never get enough of, it's beans. These perfect green-light foods are high in protein and fibre and can supplement nearly

every meal. Make bean salads or just add beans to any salad. Add to soups, replace some of the meat in casseroles or add to meat loaf. Use as a side vegetable or as an alternative to potatoes, rice or pasta. Check out the wide range of canned and frozen beans.

Exercise caution with baked beans, as the sauce can be high-fat and high-calorie. Check the label for low-fat versions and watch your serving size.

Beans have a well-deserved reputation for creating "wind," so be patient until your body adapts—as it will—to your increased consumption.

Bread	Most breads are red light except for 100% stone-ground whole wheat, or other whole grain breads with 2 1/2 to 3 grams of fibre per slice. Check labels carefully as the bread industry likes to confuse the unwary. Most bread is made from flour ground by steel rollers that strip away the bran coating, leaving a very fine powder ideal for producing light, fluffy breads and pastries. Conversely, stone-ground flour is coarser and retains more of its bran coating, so it is digested more slowly in your stomach.

Even with 100% stone-ground whole wheat bread, watch your quantity. Use very sparingly in Phase I—no more than one slice per serving.

Cereals	Use only large-flake oats, oat bran or high-fibre cold cereals (10 grams of fibre per serving or higher). Though these cereals are not much fun in themselves, you can dress up with fruit (fresh, frozen or canned), nonfat fruit-flavoured yogurt with sugar substitute, or even fruit spreads. This way you can change the menu daily. Use sweetener, not sugar.
Cottage cheese	Fat-free or 1% cottage cheese is an excellent low-fat, high-protein food. Add fruit for a snack or add it to salads.
Eggs	By far the best options are egg whites or eggs in liquid form (packaged in a carton), such as Break Free and Omega Pro. In Phase II, if you'd rather use whole eggs, buy the omega-3 kind.
Fish/Shellfish	An ideal green-light food, low in fat and cholesterol and a good source of protein. Some cold-water fish, such as salmon, are also rich in omega-3. Never eat battered or breaded fish.
Food bars	Most food or nutrition bars are a dietary disaster, high in carbohydrates and calories but low in protein. These bars are quick sugar fixes on the run. There are a few, such as Balance and Zone bars, that have a more equitable distribution of carbohydrates, proteins and fats. Look for 20 to 30 grams of carbohydrates, 10 to 15 grams of protein and 4 to 6 grams of fat. This equals about 220 calories per bar.

The serving size for a snack is one-half of a bar. Keep one in your office desk or your purse for a convenient on-the-run snack. In an emergency, I have been known to have one bar plus an apple and a glass of skim milk for lunch when a proper lunch break was impossible. This is okay in emergencies, but don't make a habit of it.

Grapefruit	One of the top-rated green-light foods. Eat as often as you like.
Hamburgers	These are acceptable but only with extra-lean ground beef that has 10 percent or less fat. Mix in some oat bran to reduce the meat content but keep the bulk. A better option would be to replace the beef with ground turkey or chicken breast. Keep the serving size at 4 ounces; use only half of a whole wheat bun and eat open-faced.
Ice Cream	Look for low-fat, no-added-sugar varieties, with 90 to 100 calories per 1/2-cup serving. And stick to this maximum serving size despite the temptation!
Milk	Use skim only. If you have trouble adjusting, then use 1% and slowly wean yourself off it. The fat you're giving up is saturated (bad) fat. Milk is a terrific snack or meal supplement. I drink two glasses of skim milk a day, at breakfast and lunch. Plain, low-fat soy milk is a great alternative.
Nuts	A principal source of "good" fat, which is essential for your health. Sliced almonds are your best choice. Add them to cereals, salads and desserts.

Oat bran An excellent high-fibre additive to baking as a partial replacement for flour. Also great as a hot cereal.

Oatmeal If you haven't had oatmeal since you were a kid, now's the time to revisit it. Large-flake or old-fashioned oatmeal is the breakfast of choice, with the added advantage for your heart of lowering cholesterol. I have had more e-mails from people describing their delight in rediscovering oatmeal than about any other single food.

Personally, I often have an oatmeal porridge snack with unsweetened applesauce and sugar substitute on the weekends. In this case, I use 1/3 cup of oats.

Oranges Fresh oranges are excellent as snacks, on cereal and especially at breakfast. A glass of orange juice has two and a half times as many calories as a whole orange, so avoid the juice and stick with the real thing.

Pasta There are two golden rules. First, do not overcook; *al dente* (some firmness to the bite) is important. Second, serving size is key: pasta is a side dish and should never occupy more than a quarter of your plate. It *must not* form the basis of the meal, as it most commonly does nowadays in North America, with disastrous results for waistlines and hips. Whole wheat pastas are preferable.

Peaches/pears Terrific snacks, desserts or additions to breakfast cereal. Use fresh, or canned in juice or water (not syrup).

Potatoes	The only form of potatoes that is acceptable even on an occasional basis is boiled new potatoes. New potatoes have a low starch content, unlike larger, more mature potatoes that have been allowed to build their starch levels. All other forms of potato—baked, mashed or fried— are strictly red light. Limit quantity to two or three per serving.
Rice	There is a wide range in the G.I. ratings for various types of rice, most of which are red light. The best rice is basmati or long grain, which is readily available at your supermarket. Brown is better than white. If rice is sticky, with the grains clumping together, don't eat it. Similarly, don't overcook rice; the more it's cooked, the more glutinous and therefore unacceptable it becomes. The rule, then, is eat only slightly undercooked basmati rice.
Salads	Try to start every dinner with a green salad. Not only will it provide an important fibre and low-G.I. nutritional boost to your meal, but it will help you feel satiated. Because acid slows the digestive process, thereby reducing the G.I. rating of the food, a vinaigrette makes an excellent accompaniment.
Soups	Canned soups have a higher G.I. rating than homemade ones because of the high temperature at which commercial varieties are processed. I have included some brands of canned soup in the green-light category because these are the best alternatives available. Homemade soups are even more green-light.

Sour Cream   One percent or nonfat sour cream with a little
sweetener stirred in is an ideal alternative to
whipped cream as a dessert topping. You can also
mix fruit or double-fruit, low-sugar fruit spread
into it for a creamy dessert.

Soy   Soy protein powder is a simple way to boost the
protein level of any meal. It's particularly useful at
breakfast for sprinkling over cereal. Look for the
kind that has a 90 percent protein content. It's
sometimes labelled "isolated soy protein powder."
Unflavoured low-fat or nonfat soy milk is a perfect
green-light beverage.

Sugar substitutes There has been a tremendous amount of misinformation circulating about artificial sweeteners—all
of which has proven groundless. The sugar industry rightly saw these new products as a threat and
has done its best to bad-mouth them. Use sweeteners such as Equal, Splenda, Sweet'N Low and
Sugar Twin to replace sugar wherever possible. If
you are allergic to sweeteners, then fructose is a
better alternative than sugar. For a medical
overview, read about sugar substitutes on the U.S.
Food and Drug Administration's Web site,
www.fda.gov.

Tofu   Though not flavourful in itself, tofu can be spiced
up in a variety of ways and is an excellent low-fat
source of protein. Use it to boost or replace meat
and seafood in stir-fries, burgers and salads.

Yogurt	Nonfat, fruit-flavoured yogurt sweetened with sugar substitute is a near-perfect green-light product. It's an ideal snack food on its own, or a flavourful addition to breakfast cereal—especially porridge—and to fruit for dessert. Our fridge is always full of it, in half a dozen delicious flavours. In fact, my shopping cart is so full of yogurt containers that fellow shoppers frequently stop me to ask if they are on special!
Yogurt Cheese	A wonderful substitute for cream in desserts or in main dishes like chili (see recipe on page 105).

Dear Rick,

I bought a beautiful red suit with thoughts of my 50th high school reunion in mind, and when it turned out to be a little snug I decided not to send it back, but to finally start the G.I. Diet and see what would happen. Since April I have lost 24 pounds, and the weight keeps coming off. I now have to take the suit in to be altered . . . My greatest dessert idea: Naval orange sections or frozen strawberries or peaches rolled in Splenda . . . I am proud of my commitment to your easy diet. Thanks for everything.

Sandie

CHAPTER SIX

Meal Ideas

When I wrote the first draft of this book, I neglected to include any recipes. My wife read the manuscript and suggested that readers would find some recipes useful, especially when getting started on the diet. Since following the G.I. Diet requires you to change how you normally eat, she felt that including recipes would demonstrate how you might adapt your own favourites to make them green-light. She suggested that my lack of enthusiasm for including recipes had more to do with my own culinary incompetence than with any pedagogical stratagems (quite true).

So, stung to action and under her direction, I decided to offer recipes for the three primary meals and snacks for Phase I of the G.I. Diet. I have tried to adapt meals that are commonly eaten by most of us, so there is no need to worry about the unfamiliar. In these recipes I have not only used green-light foods but also kept the use of fats in cooking down to a minimum. Always cook in nonstick pans, since they allow you to use only a small amount of fat when preparing food. Use a teaspoon or two of either canola or olive oil, or even better, use a vegetable oil cooking spray. Remember, there are 2,000 calories in 1 cup of oil, and fat in meat is high in cholesterol. Thus grilling and broiling are excellent ways of cooking meat, since the fat from the meat drops into the pan or onto the coals.

Cutting fat doesn't mean you have to cut flavour or lose that all-important taste sensation. Cream can be replaced with yogurt, yogurt cheese (see page 105) or nonfat sour cream. Use fat-free mayonnaise in tuna or chicken salads. You can still eat cheese, especially the strongly flavoured ones, *but sprinkle it sparingly as a flavour enhancer only*, rather than use it as the prime ingredient. Try some new spices and flavoured vinegars. Salsa will spice up many foods without adding calories or fat, and ginger adds life to stir-fries.

Breakfast

The first meal of the day is an important one, and oatmeal is the king of breakfast food. It is low-G.I. and low-calorie, is easy to prepare in the microwave, and stays with you all morning. Always use old-fashioned rolled oats—not one-minute or instant oats, as they have already been considerably processed. The body has to work harder to metabolize rolled oats, and this slows the digestive process and leaves you feeling fuller longer.

Oatmeal can be endlessly varied by changing the flavour of the fruit yogurt you add or by mixing in sliced fruit or berries. My wife's favourite way to eat oatmeal is with skim milk, unsweetened applesauce, sliced almonds and sweetener. Here's a recipe for my favourite oatmeal. Top it off with an orange and a glass of skim milk and you have a delicious breakfast that will stay with you all morning.

OATMEAL

1 serving

½ cup	old-fashioned rolled oats
1 cup	water or skim milk
½ to ¾ cup	nonfat fruit yogurt with sugar substitute
2 tbsp	sliced almonds
	Fresh fruit

Place the oats in a microwave-safe bowl and cover with water or skim milk. Microwave the oats on medium power for 3 minutes. Mix in the yogurt, almonds and some fresh fruit.

HOMEMADE MUESLI

2 servings

1 cup	old-fashioned rolled oats
¾ cup	skim milk
¾ cup	nonfat fruit yogurt with sugar substitute
2 tbsp	sliced almonds
¾ cup	diced apple or pear, or berries
	Sweetener

Place the oats in a bowl, cover them with the milk, and let soak in the refrigerator overnight. Add the yogurt, almonds, fruit, and sweetener to taste, and mix well.

ON-THE-RUN BREAKFAST

1 serving

1 cup	sliced fresh fruit, such as apple, pear or peach
½ cup	cottage cheese (1% or fat-free)
½ cup	wheat bran, such as All Bran or Bran Buds
2 tbsp	sliced almonds
1 slice	toast, spread with 2 tsp margarine (light) and 1 tbsp double-fruit, low-sugar preserves

Place the fruit in a bowl and top with the cottage cheese, wheat bran and almonds. Serve the toast alongside.

COOKING WITH SUGAR SUBSTITUTES:
Splenda, Sugar Twin and Equal can all be substituted for sugar. These sweeteners are available in several forms: individual packets, baking granules, liquid and tablets. While packets are generally equivalent in sweetness to 2 teaspoons of sugar, the intensity of sweetness can vary depending on the brand and the form, so check the label. If you are sweetening a beverage or cereal, simply use your own taste as a guide. If you are substituting for sugar in baking, follow the instructions on the box or check the product Web site. Our preference is for sweeteners such as Splenda that measure exactly the same as sugar by volume, i.e., 1 tablespoon of sugar equals 1 tablespoon of sweetener.

BASIC OMELETTE AND VARIATIONS

1 serving

Omelettes are easy to make and you can vary them by adding any number of fresh vegetables, a little cheese and/or some meat. You'll find ingredients for a basic omelette here, along with suggestions for making Italian, Mexican, vegetarian and Western versions. Don't stop with these—using the proportions as a guide, you can add whatever green-light ingredients strike your fancy. To round out the meal, include a cup of fresh fruit and a glass of skim milk or ½ to ¼ cup of nonfat fruit yogurt with sugar substitute.

> Vegetable oil cooking spray (preferably canola or olive oil)
> ½ cup   liquid egg
> ¼ cup   skim milk

Italian Omelette

> ½ cup   sliced mushrooms
> 1 oz   grated skim mozzarella cheese
> ½ cup   tomato purée
>   Chopped fresh or dried herbs, such as
>   oregano or basil

Mexican Omelette

1 cup	chopped red and green bell pepper
½ cup	sliced mushrooms
½ cup	canned beans, drained and rinsed
	Hot sauce or chili powder, for sprinkling over the omelette (optional)

Vegetarian Omelette

1 cup	broccoli florets
½ cup	sliced mushrooms
½ cup	chopped red and green bell pepper
1 oz	grated skim-milk cheese

Western Omelette

1 cup	chopped red and green bell pepper
1	small onion, chopped
2 slices	back bacon, lean deli ham or turkey breast, chopped
	Red pepper flakes or cayenne pepper (optional) for sprinkling over the omelette

Omelette Preparation

1. Spray oil in a small nonstick skillet, then place it over medium heat.
2. Add the mushrooms, bell peppers, broccoli and/or onion (depending on which omelette you are making), and sauté until tender, about 5 minutes. Transfer the sautéed vegetables to a plate and cover with aluminium foil to keep warm.

3. Beat the eggs with the milk and pour them into the skillet over medium heat. Cook until the eggs start to firm up, then spread the appropriate vegetables, cheese, herbs, beans, and/or meat over them. Continue cooking until the eggs are done to your liking.

4. If desired, sprinkle the omelette with hot sauce, chili powder, red pepper flakes or cayenne, then serve.

Variation: Make scrambled eggs by stirring the eggs as they cook, adding any additional ingredients while the eggs are still soft.

Dear Rick,

The best thing about the G.I. Diet is I don't feel as though I'm on a diet—I am choosing food I like and trying new combinations that really leave me feeling full and not thinking about food all day . . . I've cleared my cupboards and do careful shopping lists. The only problem is my family keeps eating all my "special" food. So now I cook the same for all of us. I even went away with a few girlfriends for the weekend, and we ate out every night. I chose salads and asked for double veg—no spuds. My mates felt sorry for me, until they saw my meals and were amazed. They even said I had made better choices than them . . . I love it! It is the key to happiness: lose weight but feel full all the time on lovely grub!

Beverley

Lunch

If you are eating lunch out, refer to pages 45 to 49 for helpful tips about restaurants, take-out, and fast food options. However, brown-bagging—bringing lunch to work—is becoming an increasingly popular option. It allows you to control the ingredients and amount of fat used, and you save money at the same time. The following are a number of green-light lunch recipes that you can bag and bring to work. Just add fresh or canned fruit (in water, not syrup) for dessert and have a glass of water or (preferably) skim milk. You'll feel full and energized for the afternoon.

MIXED BEAN SALAD

2 servings

1	can (540 mL) mixed beans, drained and rinsed
½	cucumber, chopped
1	tomato, chopped
1 cup	cooked whole wheat pasta (small shells, macaroni or similar shape)
2 tbsp	chopped fresh flat-leaf parsley
1 tbsp	red wine vinegar
2 tsp	olive oil
¼ tsp	Dijon mustard
	Pinch each of salt and black pepper
	Pinch of dried herbs, such as thyme or oregano

1. Place beans in large bowl and add cucumber, tomato, pasta and parsley.
2. In small bowl, whisk together vinegar, oil, mustard, salt, pepper and thyme. Pour over salad and toss to coat.

GREEK SALAD

2 servings

2 cups	torn iceberg lettuce
½	cucumber, chopped
2	tomatoes, chopped
6	kalamata olives
½	red onion, sliced
¼ cup	crumbled feta
1 tbsp	red wine vinegar
2 tsp	extra-virgin olive oil
1 tsp	fresh lemon juice
¼ tsp	dried oregano
	Pinch each of salt and black pepper

1. In bowl, toss together lettuce, cucumber, tomatoes, red onion, olives and crumbled feta.
2. In small bowl, whisk together vinegar, oil, lemon juice, oregano and salt and pepper. Pour dressing over greens and toss.

WALDORF CHICKEN AND RICE SALAD

1 serving

³/₄ cup	cooked basmati or brown rice
1	medium apple, chopped
1 or 2	stalks celery, chopped
¼ cup	walnuts
4 oz	cooked chicken (page 97), chopped
1 tbsp	store-bought light buttermilk dressing.

Place the rice, apple, celery, walnuts and chicken in a bowl. Pour the buttermilk dressing on top and stir to mix. Keep refrigerated until lunch time and enjoy.

BASIC PASTA SALAD LUNCH

1 serving

½ to ³/₄ cup	cooked whole wheat pasta (spirals, shells or similar shape)
1 cup	chopped cooked vegetables (such as broccoli, asparagus, bell peppers or green onions)
¼ cup	light tomato sauce or other low-fat or nonfat pasta sauce
4 oz	chopped cooked chicken (page 97) or other lean meat, such as ground lean turkey or lean chicken sausage

Place the pasta, vegetables, tomato sauce and chicken in a bowl and stir to mix well. Refrigerate the salad, covered, until ready to use, then heat it in the microwave or serve chilled.

Variation: You can use the proportions here as a guide and vary the vegetables, sauce and source of protein to suit your tastes and add variety to your pasta salad lunches.

COTTAGE CHEESE AND FRUIT

1 serving

Perfect for a lunch on the run.

1 cup	low-fat cottage cheese
1 cup	chopped fresh fruit or fruit canned in juice, such as peaches, apricots or pears

Place the cottage cheese and fruit in a plastic bowl with a fitted lid, and stir to mix. Store in the refrigerator until lunchtime. Enjoy.

Variation: Add a tablespoon of double-fruit, low-sugar preserves instead of the chopped fruit.

Sandwiches

The variations are endless, but here are some guidelines to make even the humble sandwich a convenient and filling green-light meal.

1. Always use 100 percent, stone-ground whole wheat or high-fibre bread.
2. During Phase 1, sandwiches should be served open faced.
3. Include at least three vegetables, such as lettuce, tomato, red or green bell pepper, cucumber, sprouts or onion.
4. Use mustard or hummus as a spread on the bread. No regular mayonnaise or butter.
5. Add 4 ounces of cooked lean meat or fish.
6. Mix tuna or chopped cooked chicken with low-fat mayonnaise or salad dressing and celery.
7. Mix canned salmon with malt vinegar (don't worry about the bones).
8. To help sandwiches stay fresh, not soggy, pack the components separately and assemble them just before eating, if possible.

Dinner

All of the following meal ideas are based on the G.I. Diet portion ratios discussed in chapter 3. Vegetables should take up 50 percent of your plate and should always comprise at least one green vegetable, a mixture of at least two other vegetables and a green salad. Meat, poultry or fish should fill 25 percent of your plate, and rice, pasta or potatoes should cover the remaining 25 percent.

I have based the following meal ideas on typical family needs, modifying them along G.I. principles.

POULTRY: BASIC PREPARATION

1 serving

Naturally low in fat, cooked chicken or turkey breast can be used in dozens of ways, combined with a variety of herbs, spices, and vegetables to enhance its flavour. You'll find instructions for a basic green-light method of cooking poultry here, followed by three recipes that use the cooked meat. The proportions are for one serving and can be multiplied as necessary for the recipes that follow.

	Vegetable oil cooking spray (preferably canola or olive oil)
4 oz	skinless, boneless chicken breast or turkey breast, whole, sliced, or cubed

1. Spray oil in a small nonstick fry pan, and then place it over medium-high heat.
2. Add the chicken or turkey breast and sauté until firm to the touch and no longer pink, about 4 minutes per side for 1 chicken breast or piece of turkey, or 5 to 6 minutes for slices or cubes.

ASIAN STIR-FRY

2 servings

	Vegetable oil cooking spray (preferably canola or olive oil)
3 cups	chopped mixed vegetables, such as carrots, cauliflower, broccoli, mushrooms and snow peas (see Note on next page)
1 tsp	grated fresh ginger
1 tsp	soy sauce
	Salt and black pepper
8 oz	cooked skinless, boneless chicken breast or turkey breast (page 97)

1. Spray oil in a nonstick skillet, then place it over medium heat.
2. Add the mixed vegetables and sauté until tender, about 5 minutes.
3. Add the ginger and soy sauce and stir to mix. Season to taste with salt and pepper.
4. Add the cooked chicken or turkey and stir to mix. Let simmer until the chicken or turkey is heated through, 2 minutes, then serve.

Variation: To put the stir-fry together even more quickly, use 2 to 3 teaspoons of a light, store-bought stir-fry sauce in place of the fresh ginger, soy sauce and salt and pepper.

Note: For convenience, use frozen mixed vegetables or frozen cut peppers.

ITALIAN CHICKEN

2 servings

8 oz	sliced mushrooms
1	medium onion, sliced
1	can (540 mL) chopped Italian tomatoes
1	clove garlic, minced
	Chopped fresh or dried oregano and basil
8 oz	cooked skinless, boneless chicken breast or turkey breast (page 97)

1. Place the mushrooms, onion and tomatoes in a saucepan. Stir in a little water, to prevent the tomatoes from sticking, and heat over medium-low heat until the mushrooms and onion are softened.
2. Add the garlic, oregano and basil, stir to mix, then let simmer for 5 minutes.
3. Add the cooked chicken or turkey and stir to mix. Let simmer until the chicken or turkey is heated through, 2 minutes, then serve.

CHICKEN CURRY

2 servings

	Vegetable oil cooking spray (preferably canola or olive oil)
1	medium onion, sliced
1 to 2 tbsp	curry powder, or more to taste
1 cup	sliced carrots
1 cup	chopped celery
½ cup	uncooked basmati rice
1	medium apple, chopped
¼ cup	raisins
4 oz	cooked skinless, boneless chicken breast or turkey breast (page 97)

1. Spray oil in a nonstick skillet, then place it over medium heat.
2. Add the onion and curry powder, stir to coat the onion with the curry, then sauté for 1 minute.
3. Add the carrots and celery, stir to mix, then sauté for 1 minute.
4. Add the rice, apple, raisins and 1 cup of water and stir to mix. Cover the skillet and let the curry simmer until all of the liquid is absorbed.
5. Add the cooked chicken or turkey and stir to mix. Keep over heat until the chicken or turkey is heated through, 2 minutes, then serve.

FISH: BASIC PREPARATION

1 serving

Virtually any fish is suitable, but *never* use commercially breaded or battered versions. Salmon and trout are great favourites in our house. Pre-spiced or flavoured varieties are okay, but why pay someone else a whopping premium for what you can easily do yourself?

Here are directions for cooking fish fillets in a microwave oven. It couldn't be easier. Proportions are for one serving and can be multiplied as necessary.

1	fish fillet (4 oz)
1 to 2 tsp	fresh lemon juice
	Black pepper

1. Place the fish fillet in a microwave-safe dish.

2. Sprinkle the lemon juice and a dash of pepper over the fish.

3. Cover the dish with microwave-safe plastic wrap, folding back one corner slightly to allow the steam to escape.

4. Microwave the fish on high power until it is opaque in colour and flakes when a fork is inserted, 4 to 5 minutes. Let stand for 2 minutes, then serve.

Variations

- Sprinkle the fish with fresh or dried herbs, such as dill, parsley, basil or tarragon.

- Cook fish on a bed of leeks and onions. (Do not add oil.)

- Sprinkle the fish with a mixture of whole wheat bread crumbs and chopped parsley (1 tablespoon per fillet) plus 1 teaspoon of melted light nonhydrogenated margarine.

A Green Light for Side Dishes

Need some ideas for what to serve alongside poultry, fish or meat? Here are a few easy-to-prepare side dishes that will fit right in with the G.I. Diet.

- Green beans with almonds or mushrooms

- Mixed vegetables, such as sliced carrots, broccoli or cauliflower florets, and halved Brussels sprouts

- Boiled new potatoes (2 to 3 per serving), tossed with herbs and a smidgen of olive oil

- Basmati rice. (You can stir some extra vegetables into the rice during the last minute of cooking.) Limit serving size to 3 tablespoons uncooked rice, which will give you ⅔ of a cup when cooked, covering a quarter of the plate.

- Pasta—about 1¼ ounces, or 35 grams, uncooked, for ¼ cup cooked, covering a quarter of the plate.

Meat

Veal and lean deli ham are your best choices. Red meat in general is a yellow-light food, although for pragmatic reasons I've included lean cuts of beef and extra-lean ground beef in Phase I. Pork and lamb tend to have a higher fat content and should be avoided until Phase II. Serving size is critical. Remember, use the palm of your hand or a pack of playing cards as a guide to portion size. And please do not be alarmed by the apparent modest size of these portions. I had a real problem downsizing my steak at first, but now my stomach reels at the portions served in many restaurants.

Steak Dinner

For a complete steak dinner, try the following:

- Broil or barbecue a fully trimmed top or eye round steak (4 ounces per person).

- Sauté sliced onions and mushrooms with a little water in a nonstick skillet, and serve with steak.

- Season chopped broccoli, asparagus, and halved Brussels sprouts with nutmeg and pepper, then microwave on high power until tender, 3 to 5 minutes.

- Boil 3 tablespoons uncooked basmati rice, or two to three new potatoes per person. Season the cooked potatoes with herbs and a touch of olive oil.

CHILI

4 servings

2 tsp	olive oil
1	large onion, sliced
2	cloves of garlic, minced
½ lb	extra-lean ground beef (optional)
2	green bell peppers, chopped
2 cups	canned tomatoes
	Chili powder to taste
½ tsp	cayenne pepper (optional)
½ tsp	salt
¼ tsp	basil
2 cups	water
1	can (540 mL) red kidney beans, drained and rinsed
1	can (540 mL) white beans, drained and rinsed Chopped tomato, chopped fresh parsley and cilantro, and/or yogurt cheese (see page 105) for garnish (optional)

1. Heal the olive oil in a deep skillet or saucepan over medium heat. Add the onion and garlic and sauté until nearly tender.
2. Add the ground beef, if using, and cook until browned, breaking up the chunks with a spoon. Drain off any fat.
3. Add the bell peppers, tomatoes, chili powder, cayenne, if using, salt, basil and water and bring to a boil. Lower the heat and let simmer, uncovered, until

the chili has reached the desired consistency, about 45 minutes.

4. Add the red and white kidney beans and cook over medium-low heat until heated through, about 5 minutes. Garnish the chili with tomato, parsley, cilantro and/or yogurt cheese if desired.

Yogurt Cheese

Looking for a green-light alternative to sour cream? Try yogurt cheese—it's easy to make your own from plain nonfat yogurt. Place a sieve lined with cheesecloth or paper towels on top of a bowl. Spoon the yogurt into the sieve and cover it with plastic wrap. Place the sieve and bowl in the refrigerator. Let the yogurt drain overnight— the next day you will have yogurt cheese.

MEAT LOAF

6 servings

1 ½ lbs	extra-lean ground beef (less than 10 percent fat)
1 cup	tomato juice
½ cup	old-fashioned rolled oats (uncooked)
1	egg, lightly beaten
½ cup	chopped onion
1 tbsp	Worcestershire sauce
½ tsp	salt (optional)
¼ tsp	black pepper

1. Preheat the oven to 350°F.

2. In a large bowl, combine all ingredients. Mix lightly but thoroughly.

3. Press the meat loaf mixture into an 8- by 4-inch loaf pan.

4. Bake the meat loaf for 1 hour, or until an instant-read meat thermometer inserted into the centre registers 160°F.

5. Let the meat loaf stand for 5 minutes before draining off any juices and slicing it.

Variation: Extra-lean ground beef is still relatively high in fat. A lower-fat and better alternative to ground beef is an equal amount of ground turkey or chicken breast. When fully cooked, ground turkey or chicken will register 170°F on an instant-read meat thermometer.

Snacks

Snacks play a critical role between meals, giving you a boost when you need it most. Have three a day: mid-morning, mid-afternoon and before bed. Most popular snack foods are disastrous from a sugar and fat standpoint. Commercial cookies, muffins and candy bars should be avoided at all costs. Fortunately, there are equally satisfying alternatives that are both convenient and low cost. Never leave home without them.

Below is a list of green-light snacks that require no preparation on your part

- 1 apple, pear, peach or orange with a few almonds
- 4 ounces low-fat cottage cheese (1% or less) mixed with 1 teaspoon low-sugar, double fruit preserves
- ¾ cup nonfat fruit yogurt with sugar substitute
- ½ of a food bar such as Balance or Zone (200 calories; 20 to 30 grams carbohydrates; 12 to 15 grams protein; and 5 grams fat per bar)
- 8 to 10 almonds, hazelnuts or peanuts

You will find several other easy-to-make snack recipes in chapter 8.

CHAPTER SEVEN

Phase II

Congratulations! You've achieved your new weight target!

Now is the moment to go back to page 34 and complete the chart you started a few months ago. Compare what you ate then with your current diet. I promise you'll be amazed at the change.

This may be hard to believe, but when I had reached my target weight—I had lost 22 pounds, and 3 inches off my waist—I had to make a conscious effort to eat more in order to avoid losing more weight. My wife said I was entering the "gaunt zone"!

Phase II Meals and Snacks

The objective in Phase II is to increase the number of calories you consume so that you maintain your new weight. Remember the equation: food energy ingested must equal energy expended to keep weight stable. During Phase I you were taking in less food energy than you were expending, using your fat reserves to make up the short-fall. Now we make up that deficit by taking in some extra food energy, or calories.

Two words of caution. First, your body has become accustomed to doing with fewer calories and has, to a certain extent, adapted. The result is that your body is more efficient than in the bad old days when it had more food energy than it could use. Second, your new lower weight requires fewer calories to function. For example, if you lost 10 percent of your weight, then you need 10 percent fewer calories for your body to function.

Combining a more efficient body, which requires less energy to operate, with a lower weight, which requires fewer calories, means that you need only a marginal increase in food energy to balance the energy in/energy out equation. The biggest mistake most people make when coming off a diet is assuming that they can now consume a much higher calorie level than their new body really needs. The bottom line is that Phase II is only marginally different from Phase I. Phase II provides you with an opportunity to make small adjustments to portion size and add new foods from the yellow-light category. All the fundamentals of the Phase I plan, however, remain inviolable. The following are some suggestions for how you might wish to modify your new eating pattern in Phase II:

Breakfast

- Increase cereal serving size, e.g., from ½ to ⅔ cup oatmeal.

- Add a slice of 100% whole-grain toast and a pat of margarine.

- Double up on the sliced almonds on cereals.

- Help yourself to an extra slice of back bacon.

- Have a glass of juice now and then.

- Add one of the forbidden fruits—a banana or apricots—to your cereal.

- Have a fully caffeinated coffee. Try to limit yourself to one a day, and make sure it's a good one!

Lunch

I suggest you continue to eat lunch as you did in Phase I. This is the one meal that contained some compromises in the weight-loss portion of the program, since it is a meal most of us buy each day.

Dinner

- Add another boiled new potato (from two or three to three or four).

- Increase the rice or pasta serving from ¼ to 1 cup.

- Have a 6-ounce steak instead of your regular 4 ounce. Make this a special treat, not a habit.

- Eat a few more olives and nuts, but watch the serving size as these are calorie heavyweights.

- Try a cob of sweet corn with a dab of nonhydrogenated margarine.

- Add a slice of whole-grain, high-fibre bread.

- Have a lean cut of lamb or pork (maximum 4-ounce serving).

- Have a glass of red wine with dinner.

Snacks

WARNING: Strictly watch quantity or serving size.

- Light microwave popcorn (maximum 2 cups)

- Nuts, maximum eight to ten

- A square or two of bittersweet chocolate (see next page)

- A banana

- One scoop of low-fat ice cream

Chocolate

To many of us, the idea of a chocolate-free world is abhorrent. The good news is that some chocolate, in limited quantities, is acceptable.

Most chocolate contains large quantities of saturated fat and sugar, making it quite fattening. However, chocolate with a high cocoa content (70 percent) delivers more chocolate satisfaction per ounce. So, a square or two of rich, dark, bittersweet chocolate, nibbled slowly or, better yet, dissolved in the mouth, gives us chocoholics just the fix we need. This high-cocoa chocolate is available at specialty stores and can be found in many supermarkets.

Alcohol

Now is the moment some of you have been waiting for. In Phase II a daily glass of wine, preferably red and with dinner, is not only allowed—it's encouraged! Recently, there has been a flood of research into the benefits of alcohol on personal health. It is generally agreed that some alcohol is better than none at all, especially for heart health. It has been found that red wine in particular is rich in flavonoids and, when drunk in moderation (a glass a day), has a demonstrable benefit in reducing the risk of heart attack and stroke. The theory that says if one glass is good for you, two must be better is tempting but not true. One glass gives the optimum benefit.

As with coffee, if you're only going to have a glass of wine a day, make it a great one. My eldest son, who is a computer programmer in Seattle and lives a lifestyle I can only dream about, took me at my word about wine and gave me a subscription to the *Wine Spectator*. It has proven to be the most costly present I've ever received, as a whole new world of wine and wine ratings has opened up to me. My $10-a-bottle ceiling for special occasions has now doubled or tripled, though it has all been rationalized: I'm drinking less, so I can afford the extravagance!

As a beer aficionado, I like to drink the occasional beer as an alternative to wine. This habit has recently received an endorsement from a group of scientists who reported in late 1999 that beer (in moderation) would reduce cholesterol and thus heart disease, delay menopause, and reduce the risk of several cancers. They also noted that beer has anti-inflammatory and anti-allergic properties, plus a positive effect on bone density. Personally, I worry about any product being touted as the wonder cure for all our ills, but clearly a glass of beer with supper is likely to do more good than harm. Remember, though, that because of its high malt content, beer is a high-G.I. beverage, so moderation is particularly important.

If you do drink alcohol, always have it with your meal. Food slows down the absorption of alcohol, thereby minimizing its impact.

The Way You Will Eat for the Rest of Your Life

With all these new options in Phase II, the temptation may be to overdo it. If the pounds start to reappear, simply revert to the Phase I plan for a while and you'll be astonished at how quickly your equilibrium is restored.

Phase II is the way you will eat for the rest of your life. You will look and feel better, have more energy and experience none of those hypoglycemic lows. One reason, of course, that you have more energy is that you're not carrying around all that surplus fat. It might be fun to resurrect the backpack and load it up with the weight you've just lost. Carry it around on your back for an hour or two and then rejoice that you don't have to carry it around for the rest of your life! Whenever your resolve wavers, reach for the backpack. It's a marvellous motivator.

The opportunity to succeed is in your hands. I've tried to give you a simple yet motivating plan that will not leave you hungry, tired or confused. It's all here in the book; the rest is up to you.

So, put on the backpack for a couple of hours, clear out the pantry and drive to the supermarket. Remember to park as far as possible from the entrance and enjoy the extra walk. Everything starts with a first step!

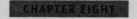

CHAPTER EIGHT

Recipes

Breakfast

HUEVOS RANCHEROS   GREEN-LIGHT

These eggs are a spicy way to start the day and are very filling. They are poached to perfection in the oven, so you can enjoy your guests while brunch cooks away.

2 tsp	canola oil
1	onion, chopped
2	cloves garlic, minced
1	small jalapeño pepper, minced
1 tbsp	chili powder
1 tsp	dried oregano
1 tsp	ground cumin
1	can (398 mL) stewed tomatoes
1 cup	vegetable cocktail or tomato juice
1	can (540 mL) black beans, drained and rinsed
1	can (540 mL) chickpeas, drained and rinsed
1	green bell pepper, finely chopped
¼ cup	chopped fresh cilantro
2 tbsp	chopped fresh flat-leaf parsley
6	eggs
6	small whole wheat tortillas

1. Heat the oil over medium heat in a large nonstick skillet and cook the onion, garlic, jalapeño pepper, chili powder, oregano and cumin until the onion starts to soften, about 3 minutes. Add the tomatoes, vegetable

juice, black beans, chickpeas, green pepper, and half each of the cilantro and parsley, and bring to a boil. Reduce the heat and simmer until slightly thickened, about 15 minutes. Pour the mixture into a 9 x 13-inch baking dish.

2. Preheat the oven to 425°F.

3. Break 1 egg into a small bowl and carefully slide it onto the bean mixture. Repeat with the remaining eggs, spacing them out like cookies on a baking sheet. Cover the dish with aluminum foil and bake until the whites of the eggs are set (or longer if desired), about 10 minutes. Sprinkle the remaining cilantro and parsley over the dish and serve with tortillas.

Makes 6 servings.

SOUTHWEST OMELETTE ROLL-UP   `GREEN-LIGHT`

Brunch is a great time to gather with friends and family, but you don't want to spend all your time at the stove. Here is a family-size omelette with a southwest bean filling that you can make ahead of time. It's perfect with a salad and fresh fruit.

Roux:

2 tbsp	canola oil
3 tbsp	whole wheat flour
1 cup	warm skim milk
¼ tsp	salt
	Pinch of black pepper
	Pinch of ground cumin (optional)

Omelette:

4	egg whites
1 cup	liquid egg

Filling:

1	package (250 g) light cream cheese, softened
½ cup	low-fat salsa
1	can (540 mL) red kidney beans or black beans, drained and rinsed
1	red or green bell pepper, diced
2	green onions, sliced
¼ cup	chopped fresh cilantro or flat-leaf parsley

1. **Make the roux:** Heat the oil in a small saucepan over medium heat and add the flour. Cook for 1 minute,

whisking constantly. Slowly add the milk and cook, whisking gently, until thick enough to coat the back of a spoon, about 5 minutes. Whisk in the salt, pepper and cumin, if using, and whisk to combine thoroughly. Pour into a large bowl and let cool.

2. Preheat the oven to 350°F. Grease an 11 x 17-inch baking sheet and line it with parchment paper.

3. Meanwhile, in another bowl, beat the egg whites to stiff peaks. Whisk the liquid egg into the roux and fold half of the egg whites into the mixture. Add the remaining egg whites, folding gently until combined. Pour the mixture onto the prepared baking sheet. Bake until the eggs are puffed, lightly golden, and firm to the touch, about 18 minutes. Let cool on the baking sheet.

4. **Make the filling:** Combine the cream cheese and salsa in a large bowl and stir until smooth. Stir in the beans, red pepper, green onions and cilantro and set aside.

5. Run a small knife around the edges of the baking sheet and place a clean tea towel over the top. Invert the eggs onto a work surface and gently peel off the parchment paper. Spread the filling evenly over the eggs, leaving a 2-inch border on one of the long sides.

6. Using the tea towel as a guide, roll up the omelette starting with the other long side and working toward the long side with the 2-inch border. Cut in half to make 2 rolls. Using a long spatula or palette knife, transfer the rolls to a large serving platter. Cut each roll into 4 pieces before serving.

Makes 8 servings.

GREEN EGGS AND HAM

`GREEN-LIGHT`

A beloved childhood story comes to life, with very healthy results. Spinach adds colour and flavour to the egg mixture, and lean ham adds a salty zing. This is a recipe that begs to be shared with family and friends at a festive breakfast.

1 tsp	canola oil
1	small onion, finely diced
1	clove garlic, minced
2	red bell peppers, thinly sliced
¼ cup	chopped fresh flat-leaf parsley
¼ tsp	dried basil or marjoram, or 1 tsp chopped fresh
1 tbsp	Dijon mustard
6 slices	lean ham or back bacon

Green Eggs:

1	bag (300 g) baby spinach
1 tsp	canola oil
2 cups	liquid egg
½ tsp	salt
¼ tsp	black pepper
2 tbsp	chopped fresh flat-leaf parsley
2 tbsp	chopped fresh basil

1. Heat the oil in a nonstick skillet over medium heat. Add the onion and garlic and cook for 3 minutes. Add the peppers, parsley and basil and cook until the

peppers are tender-crisp, about 3 minutes. Scrape the mixture into a 9 x 13-inch baking dish.

2. Spread each ham slice with some of the mustard and place the slices on top of the pepper mixture in a layer. Set aside.

3. **Make the Green Eggs:** Rinse the spinach in a colander and let drain. Heat a large nonstick skillet over medium-high heat. Add the spinach, in batches if necessary; cover; and cook until bright green and wilted, about 3 minutes. Drain again, let cool somewhat, and squeeze any excess water out. Chop the spinach and set it aside.

4. Preheat the oven to 400°F.

5. Heat the oil in a nonstick skillet over medium heat. Meanwhile, whisk together in a large bowl the liquid egg, salt and pepper. Add the chopped spinach and stir to combine.

6. Pour the spinach-egg mixture into the skillet and cook, without stirring, until the mixture begins to set around the edges. Lift one of the edges with a spatula and tilt the pan so the uncooked portion flows underneath. Sprinkle the parsley and basil over the eggs and continue cooking until the eggs are just set.

7. Cut the eggs into six portions and spoon one portion of the cooked eggs onto each of the ham slices. Cover the dish with aluminum foil and bake for about 10 minutes to warm through.

Makes 6 servings.

Soups

CREAM OF SPINACH SOUP   `GREEN-LIGHT`

Many creamed soups contain, as their names suggest, cream. Some others get a creamy texture from the addition of puréed potatoes. This soup calls for puréed white beans, which add fibre, flavour and creaminess while keeping it green-light.

1 tsp	canola oil
1	onion, chopped
1	stalk celery, chopped
1	carrot, chopped
2	cloves garlic, minced
1 tbsp	chopped fresh thyme, or 1 tsp dried
2	tomatoes, chopped
5 cups	vegetable or chicken broth (low-fat, low-sodium)
1	can (540 mL) white kidney beans, drained and rinsed
1	bag (300 g) baby spinach, trimmed
	Pinch each of salt and black pepper

1. Heat the oil in a soup pot over medium heat. Add the onion, celery, carrot, garlic and thyme and cook until the onion has softened, about 5 minutes. Add the tomatoes and cook for 2 minutes. Add the vegetable broth and beans and bring to a boil. Reduce the heat and simmer for 10 minutes.

2. Meanwhile, using a chef's knife, finely chop the spinach, then set it aside.
3. Working in batches, purée the soup in a blender until smooth, then return the soup to the pot. Bring to a gentle boil and add the spinach, salt and pepper. Cook, stirring, until the spinach is tender, wilted and bright green, about 5 minutes.

Makes 4 to 6 servings.

CAULIFLOWER AND CHICKPEA SOUP   GREEN-LIGHT

This combination will help you find another reason to buy cauliflower again—it's absolutely delicious with a hint of ginger and cumin.

1 tsp	canola oil
1	onion, peeled and chopped
2	cloves garlic, minced
1	each carrot and celery stalk, chopped
1 tbsp	minced peeled ginger
2 tsp	ground cumin
½ tsp	ground coriander
¼ tsp	ground turmeric
6 cups	chopped cauliflower (see Note on next page)
2	cans (540 mL each) chickpeas, drained and rinsed
6 cups	vegetable or chicken broth (low-fat, low-sodium)
½ cup	nonfat plain yogurt
3 tbsp	chopped fresh cilantro

1. Heat the oil in a soup pot over medium heat. Add the onion, garlic, carrot, celery, ginger, cumin, coriander and turmeric and cook until the onion has softened, about 5 minutes. Add the cauliflower and chickpeas and cook, stirring, about 2 minutes. Add the vegetable broth and bring to a boil. Cover, and simmer until the cauliflower is tender, about 20 minutes.

2. Transfer the soup to a blender or food processor and, working in batches, purée until smooth. Return the soup to the pot and reheat. Serve with a dollop of yogurt and a sprinkle of cilantro.

Makes 6 to 8 servings.

Storage: Once the soup is completely cool you can store it in airtight containers in the refrigerator for up to 3 days, or freeze it for up to 1 month.

Note: You will need to buy 1 small head of cauliflower (about 2 pounds) to get 6 cups of chopped cauliflower.

SOUTHWEST CHICKEN AND BEAN SOUP

`GREEN-LIGHT`

This has the flavour of a chicken chili but the consistency of a soup. You can make your own nacho chips to serve alongside by cutting whole-wheat pitas into 8 wedges each and toasting them on a baking sheet in a 400°F oven for 10 minutes.

1 tsp	canola oil
1	onion, finely chopped
2	cloves garlic, minced
2 tsp	chili powder
½ tsp	paprika
½ tsp	ground cumin
6 cups	chicken broth (low-fat, low-sodium)
1	can (398 mL) stewed tomatoes
1	each red and green bell pepper, diced
12 oz	boneless chicken, finely chopped
1	can (425 g) red kidney beans, drained and rinsed
2 tbsp	chopped fresh cilantro
2 tbsp	fresh lime juice

1. Heat the oil in a soup pot over medium heat. Add the onion, garlic, chili powder, paprika and cumin and cook until the onion has softened, about 5 minutes.

2. Add the chicken broth, tomatoes and red and green peppers, and bring to a boil. Reduce the heat to a gentle boil and add the chicken and beans. Cook, stirring, for about 8 minutes or until the chicken is no longer pink inside. Add the cilantro and lime juice before serving.

Makes 4 servings.

Salads

MEDITERRANEAN RICE SALAD WITH
TANGY MUSTARD HERB DRESSING   GREEN-LIGHT

Here's a great dinner whose leftovers (if there are any) are just as good the next day for lunch. Meat lovers can feel free to add sliced ham or turkey.

1 ½ cups	vegetable or chicken broth
¾ cup	brown rice
¼ tsp	salt
2 cups	lightly-packed baby spinach leaves
2 cups	shredded red-leaf lettuce
2	tomatoes, chopped
1	can (540 mL) mixed beans, drained and rinsed
1	zucchini, diced
1	red bell pepper, diced
1 cup	diced cucumber
2	hard-boiled eggs, peeled and quartered

Tangy Mustard Herb Dressing:

¼ cup	rice vinegar
2 tbsp	chopped fresh basil
2 tbsp	chopped fresh flat-leaf parsley
1 tbsp	extra-virgin olive oil
2 tsp	Dijon mustard
¼ tsp	each salt and black pepper

1. Bring the broth, rice and salt to a boil in a soup pot. Reduce the heat to low, cover, and cook until the liquid is absorbed, about 35 minutes. Remove from the heat and let stand for about 5 minutes. Fluff the rice with a fork and let cool slightly.

2. Meanwhile, put the spinach, lettuce, tomatoes, beans, zucchini, red pepper and cucumber in a large serving bowl. Add the rice and toss to combine. Scatter the egg on top.

3. **Make the Tangy Mustard Herb Dressing:** Whisk together in a small bowl the vinegar, basil, parsley, oil, mustard, salt and pepper.

4. Pour over the salad and toss gently to coat.

Makes 4 to 6 servings.

NIÇOISE SALAD
GREEN-LIGHT

Here's a salad that is a meal in itself. You can enjoy fresh grilled tuna instead of canned when available. Look for firm, bright-coloured tuna that has no fishy aroma. Grill for about 2 minutes per side for a perfect rare tuna steak.

1 lb	green beans, trimmed
2 cups	torn red-leaf lettuce
2 cups	torn Boston lettuce
4	small new potatoes, cooked
2	cans (170 g each) chunk white tuna, drained
2	hard-boiled eggs
1	can (540 mL) chickpeas, drained and rinsed
1 cup	grape tomatoes
½	small red onion, thinly sliced (optional)
¼	cup small pitted black olives

Anchovy Mustard Vinaigrette:

1	anchovy fillet, minced, or 1 tsp anchovy paste
1 tbsp	Dijon mustard
1	small clove garlic, minced
¼ cup	white wine vinegar
2 tbsp	extra-virgin olive oil
¼ tsp	salt
¼ tsp	black pepper
	Pinch of paprika
2 tbsp	chopped fresh basil or flat-leaf parsley

1. Bring a saucepan of water to a boil. Add the green beans and cook until tender-crisp, about 7 minutes. Drain them, and rinse under cold water until cool. Set aside.

2. Spread the red-leaf and Boston lettuce onto a large platter. Cut the potatoes in quarters and arrange them attractively on the lettuce. Add the cooked beans, tuna, eggs, chickpeas, tomatoes, red onion, if using, and olives.

3. **Make the Anchovy Mustard Vinaigrette:** In a bowl, mash the anchovy fillet with a fork and add the Dijon mustard and garlic. Continue to mash to combine. Whisk in the vinegar, oil, salt, pepper and paprika. Drizzle the vinaigrette over the salad platter. Sprinkle with the basil.

Makes 4 to 6 servings.

JERK PORK SALAD   YELLOW-LIGHT

Jerk is a traditional Jamaican seasoning used to spice up
pork, chicken and fish. Hot peppers give this some bite,
and herbs lend flavour that has a cooling effect.

3	green onions, chopped
1	large clove garlic, chopped
½	each green and red bell pepper, chopped
1	small scotch bonnet or jalapeno pepper, seeded
1 tbsp	chopped fresh thyme or 1 tsp dried
1 tsp	each ground allspice and nutmeg
½ tsp	black pepper
2 tbsp	fresh lime juice
1 tbsp	canola oil
2	pork tenderloins (12 oz each)

Chili Lime Vinaigrette:

2 tbsp	apple cider vinegar
2 tsp	each Dijon mustard and canola oil
½ tsp	grated lime zest
1 tbsp	fresh lime juice
½ tsp	sugar substitute
¼ tsp	chili powder
	Pinch each of salt and black pepper
6 cups	mixed baby greens
1 cup	halved grape tomatoes
1 cup	chopped cucumber
1	can (540 mL) mixed beans, drained and rinsed

1. Preheat an outdoor grill or a grill pan.
2. Combine in a food processor the green onions, garlic, green and red bell peppers, scotch bonnet pepper, thyme, allspice, nutmeg and black pepper. Pulse until a smooth paste forms. Pulse in the lime juice and oil.
3. Place the tenderloins in a shallow dish and spread with the jerk seasoning, turning to coat. Cover and refrigerate for at least 20 minutes and up to 8 hours.
4. **Make the Chili Lime Vinaigrette:** Whisk together in a small bowl the vinegar, mustard, oil, lime zest and juice, sugar substitute, chili powder, salt and black pepper.
5. Place the tenderloins on the greased grill over medium-high heat. Cook, turning occasionally, for about 20 minutes or until only a hint of pink remains. Remove to a plate.
6. In a serving bowl, toss together the baby greens, tomatoes, cucumber and mixed beans. Pour the vinaigrette over the salad and toss to coat.
7. Thinly slice the pork tenderloins and serve on top of the greens.

Makes 6 servings.

SHRIMP CAESAR SALAD　　　GREEN-LIGHT

Caesar salad is wonderful as a meal, and by adding grilled chicken breast or roasted salmon fillet you can change the flavour.

3 slices	stone-ground whole wheat bread
2 tbsp	finely chopped fresh flat-leaf parsley
2	cloves garlic, minced
2 tsp	extra-virgin olive oil
½ tsp	dried basil
	Pinch each of salt and black pepper
4 cups	chopped romaine lettuce
1	can (540 mL) mixed beans, drained and rinsed
1 cup	grape tomatoes, halved
12 oz	large cooked shrimp

Anchovy Garlic Dressing:

3	cloves garlic, minced
2	anchovy fillets, finely minced (see Hint)
2 tsp	Dijon mustard
3 tbsp	chicken broth (low-fat, low-sodium)
4 tsp	extra-virgin olive oil
1 tbsp	fresh lemon juice
¼ tsp	each salt and black pepper

1. Preheat the oven to 400°F.
2. Cut the bread into ¾-inch pieces and place them in a bowl. Add the parsley, garlic, oil, basil, salt and pepper and toss to coat well. Spread the bread onto a baking

sheet lined with parchment paper and bake until golden and crisp, about 15 minutes. Let cool.

3. In a large serving bowl, combine the lettuce, beans, tomatoes and shrimp. Set aside.

4. **Make the Anchovy Garlic Dressing:** In a small bowl, mash together with a fork the garlic, anchovies and mustard. Whisk in the chicken broth, oil, lemon juice, salt and pepper.

5. Pour the dressing over the salad and toss to coat. Sprinkle with croutons before serving.

Makes 4 servings.

Helpful Hint: You can use 2 tsp anchovy paste instead of the anchovy fillets. Look for it in the dairy section of your grocery store.

Meatless

VEGETARIAN SHEPHERD'S PIE `GREEN-LIGHT`

Here is a lighter twist on a traditionally quite heavy dish. While a traditional shepherd's pie is filled with ground beef or lamb, this one is filled instead with bulgur and beans. It's still comforting and filled with protein, just healthier. Bulgur is also sold as "Middle Eastern pasta" or cracked wheat. If you like, you can skip the potato topping and serve the pie in bowls, like chili.

1 tsp	canola oil
1	small onion, finely chopped
2	cloves garlic, minced
3/4 cup	bulgur
1 tsp	dried oregano
1/2 tsp	dried basil
1 1/2 cups	vegetable broth
1 cup	canned stewed tomatoes with juices
2	new red potatoes
1/4 cup	water
1	can (540 mL) chickpeas, drained and rinsed
1 cup	frozen peas
1/2 tsp	salt
1/2 tsp	black pepper
2 tbsp	chopped fresh flat-leaf parsley

1. Heat the oil in a nonstick skillet over medium heat. Add the onion, garlic, bulgur, oregano and basil and cook until the onion is softened, about 5 minutes. Add the broth and tomatoes, breaking up the tomatoes with the back of a spoon, and bring to a boil. Reduce the heat to simmer, cover, and cook until the bulgur is just tender, about 10 minutes.

2. Preheat the oven to 400°F.

3. Meanwhile, pierce the potatoes all over with a fork. Place the potatoes in a small bowl with the water and microwave on high for 5 minutes. Let cool.

4. Add the chickpeas, peas and half each of the salt and pepper to the bulgur mixture and stir to combine. Scrape into an 8-inch casserole dish, smoothing the top.

5. Thinly slice the potatoes and layer them, overlapping slightly, on top of the bulgur mixture. Sprinkle with the remaining salt and pepper and the parsley.

6. Bake until the mixture is bubbly, about 20 minutes. Let cool slightly before serving.

Makes 4 servings.

Helpful Hint: If you prefer not to microwave the potatoes, boil them in a saucepan filled with enough water to cover them for about 10 minutes, or until tender but firm.

BEAN AND ONION PIZZA GREEN-LIGHT

Here's a restaurant favourite that is custom-made for your G.I. lifestyle.

Pizza Dough:

³/₄ cup	warm water
2 ¹/₄ tsp	active dry yeast
1 ¹/₃ cups	whole wheat flour
¹/₂ cup	wheat bran
	Pinch of salt

Topping:

1 tsp	canola oil
2	onions, thinly sliced
2	cloves garlic, minced
¹/₄ tsp	dried thyme
	Pinch each of salt and black pepper
¹/₄ cup	sun-dried tomatoes
¹/₂ cup	boiling water
1 cup	cooked red kidney beans
³/₄ cup	low-fat pasta sauce
2 tbsp	chopped fresh basil
³/₄ cup	crumbled light feta cheese

1. **Make the Pizza Dough:** Pour the water into a large bowl and sprinkle with the yeast. Let stand for about 10 minutes or until frothy. Stir in 1¼ cups of the flour, the bran and salt until a ragged dough forms. Let stand, covered, for 30 minutes. Place the dough onto a

floured surface and knead it, adding more of the remaining flour as necessary, just until it forms a soft, slightly sticky dough. Place in a greased bowl, cover, and let rest until doubled in bulk, about 1 hour.

2. **Make the Topping:** Heat the oil in a nonstick skillet over medium-high heat. Add the onions and garlic and cook, stirring, until the onions are starting to become golden, about 3 minutes. Reduce the heat to medium and add the thyme, salt and pepper. Continue cooking, stirring occasionally, until the onions are soft and golden brown, about 15 minutes.

3. Soak the sun-dried tomatoes in the boiling water and let stand for 5 minutes. Drain and discard the water and chop the tomatoes.

4. Preheat the oven to 425°F. Punch down the dough and roll it out on a floured surface to fit a 12- to 14-inch round pizza pan. Place the dough on the pan, stretching it as necessary to fit.

5. Put the beans in a large mixing bowl and mash them with a potato masher. Stir in the pasta sauce, sun-dried tomatoes and basil. Spread the topping over the pizza dough. Top with the onions and sprinkle with feta.

6. Bake for about 20 minutes or until golden and crisp.

Makes 4 servings.

MUSHROOM AND BEAN RAGOUT   `GREEN-LIGHT`

A ragout is a thick sauce that is wonderful served over
noodles or rice. I like it served over radiatore or rotini
pasta. You can also serve it on its own, like chili.

2 tsp	extra-virgin olive oil
1 lb	mushrooms, finely chopped
1	onion, chopped
4	cloves garlic, minced
1	small stalk celery, chopped
1	small carrot, diced
1 tsp	each Italian herb seasoning and paprika
1	can (796 mL) diced tomatoes
1	can (540 mL) kidney beans, drained and rinsed
1/4 cup	tomato paste
	Pinch each of salt and black pepper

1. Heat the oil in a large, shallow Dutch oven over
   medium-high heat. Cook the mushrooms, onion, garlic, celery, carrot, Italian herb seasoning and paprika
   until the onion is golden and the liquid from the
   mushrooms evaporates, about 10 minutes.
2. Add the tomatoes, beans, tomato paste, salt and pepper
   and bring to a boil. Reduce the heat and simmer gently for about 25 minutes or until thickened.

Makes 4 servings.

WHITE BEAN MASH

GREEN-LIGHT

This creamy side dish is a higher fibre alternative to mashed potatoes. The creaminess comes from the addition of vegetable broth. Add your favourite greens like watercress for a peppery bite or kale for a heartier winter version.

1 cup	vegetable broth (low-fat, low-sodium)
2	cans (540 mL) white kidney beans, drained and rinsed
¼ tsp	dried thyme
¼ tsp	black pepper
2 cups	baby spinach leaves, shredded
	Pinch of salt

1. Bring the vegetable broth to a boil in a saucepan. Add the beans, thyme and black pepper. Simmer for about 10 minutes

2. Mash the bean mixture with a potato masher until fairly smooth. Stir in the spinach and salt until combined.

Makes 4 servings.

VEGETARIAN MOUSSAKA   GREEN-LIGHT

Traditionally made with ground lamb, moussaka can be
made low-GI by using vegetables.

2	large eggplants (about 3 lbs total)
2 tsp	salt
1 tsp	canola oil
2	large onions, finely chopped
3	cloves garlic, minced
1	each red and green bell pepper, diced
1 tbsp	dried oregano
1 tsp	ground cinnamon
1/2 tsp	black pepper
1/4 tsp	ground allspice
1	can (796 mL) diced tomatoes
1/4 cup	tomato paste
1	can (540 mL) chickpeas, drained and rinsed
1/4 cup	chopped fresh flat-leaf parsley

Cheese Sauce:

2 tbsp	canola oil
1/4 cup	whole wheat flour
2 cups	warm skim milk
1/4 tsp	salt
	Pinch each of nutmeg and black pepper
2/3 cup	liquid egg
1/2 cup	1% pressed cottage cheese
1 cup	crumbled light feta cheese

1. Preheat the oven to 425°F. Cut the eggplants into
   1/4-inch-thick slices and layer them in a colander,

sprinkling each layer with some of the salt. Let stand for 30 minutes, then rinse the slices and drain them well. Place them on baking sheets lined with parchment paper and roast, in batches if necessary, for about 20 minutes or until tender. Set aside.

2. Heat the oil in a large, shallow Dutch oven or deep nonstick skillet over medium heat. Add the onions, garlic, red and green peppers, oregano, cinnamon, pepper and allspice and cook until the onions have softened, about 5 minutes. Add the tomatoes and tomato paste and bring to a boil. Add the chickpeas and parsley, reduce the heat, and simmer for 15 minutes.

3. **Make the Cheese Sauce:** Heat the oil in a saucepan over medium heat. Stir in the flour and cook for 1 minute. Whisk in the milk and cook, whisking gently, for about 10 minutes or until the mixture is thick enough to coat the back of a spoon. Stir in the salt, nutmeg and black pepper. Let cool slightly and whisk in the egg and cottage cheese.

4. Preheat the oven to 350°F. Spread one third of the tomato sauce on the bottom of a 9 x 13-inch baking dish. Top with one third of the eggplant slices and one quarter of the feta cheese. Repeat the layers. After the last layer of eggplant, spread the cheese sauce evenly over the top and sprinkle with the remaining feta.

5. Bake for about 1 hour or until the top is golden brown. Let stand for 10 minutes before serving.

Makes 8 servings.

ROASTED VEGETABLE
MACARONI AND CHEESE   `YELLOW-LIGHT`

Macaroni and cheese is a favourite comfort food, so why not add some vegetables for flavour, colour, and fibre?

2	carrots, coarsely chopped
2	zucchini, chopped
2	cloves garlic
1	small eggplant, cubed
1	red bell pepper, chopped
1	onion, cut into 8 wedges
1/4 cup	vegetable broth (low-fat, low-sodium)
1 tsp	dried thyme
1/2 tsp	salt
1/4 tsp	black pepper

Cheese Sauce:

3 tbsp	canola oil
1/3 cup	whole wheat flour
3 cups	warm skim milk
2 tsp	Dijon mustard
1 cup	shredded light-style cheddar cheese
2 tbsp	grated Parmesan cheese
1/4 tsp	each salt and black pepper
1 1/2 cups	whole wheat macaroni

1. Preheat the oven to 425°F. Toss together in a large bowl the carrots, zucchini, garlic, eggplant, red pepper, onion, vegetable broth, thyme, salt and pepper. Spread

the mixture in a single layer on a large baking sheet lined with parchment paper or foil. Roast for about 35 minutes or until golden brown and tender-crisp. Set aside.

2. Bring a large pot of salted water to a boil.

3. **Make the Cheese Sauce:** Heat the oil in a large saucepan over medium-high heat. Add the flour and cook, stirring, for about 1 minute. Slowly whisk in the milk and continue whisking gently until the mixture is thick enough to coat the back of a spoon, about 5 minutes. Add the mustard, cheddar and Parmesan cheeses, salt and pepper and whisk until smooth. Remove from the heat.

4. Meanwhile, cook the macaroni in the boiling water until al dente, about 8 minutes. Drain well and add to the cheese sauce. Add the roasted vegetables and stir to combine.

Makes 4 to 6 servings.

Make Ahead: If you want to make this a day ahead, simply wrap the casserole dish before baking with plastic wrap and refrigerate. Remove the plastic wrap and bake in a 350°F oven for about 45 minutes or until heated through.

ROASTED PEPPER AND TOMATO STRATA

GREEN-LIGHT

Stratas are casseroles layered with bread. We've made ours green-light by using whole wheat bread and cutting back on the amount. This is a perfect make-ahead brunch or potluck dish.

8 slices	stone-ground whole wheat bread
2	jars (300 mL each) roasted red peppers, drained
4 cups	chopped cooked broccoli
1 cup	shredded light-style Swiss cheese
2 cups	skim milk
1 cup	liquid egg
2 tbsp	Dijon mustard
2 tbsp	chopped fresh flat-leaf parsley
¼ tsp	salt
¼ tsp	black pepper
2	tomatoes, sliced

1. Trim the crusts off the bread. Cut the slices into ¼-inch cubes and sprinkle half over the bottom of a greased 9 x 13-inch baking dish.
2. Slice the peppers into long, thin strips. Sprinkle half of the peppers and half of the broccoli over the bread. Sprinkle with half of the cheese. Top with the remaining bread cubes, peppers, broccoli and cheese.
3. Whisk together in a large bowl the milk, liquid egg, mustard, parsley, salt and pepper. Pour over the bread

mixture, cover, and refrigerate for at least 2 hours or up to 24 hours.

4. Preheat the oven to 350°F. Place the tomato slices on top of the casserole, overlapping slightly if necessary. Bake, uncovered, for about 45 minutes or until edges are golden and a knife inserted in the centre comes out clean.

Makes 8 to 10 servings.

Fish and Seafood

SHRIMP AND CRAB CAKES   GREEN-LIGHT

These little cakes are brunch showstoppers. You can use scallops instead of the shrimp, and baby spinach for the arugula. However you choose to make them, these will disappear before your eyes.

1	can (540 mL) chickpeas, drained and rinsed
1 lb	large raw shrimp, peeled and deveined
2 cups	crabmeat
¾ cup	fresh whole wheat bread crumbs
⅓ cup	liquid egg
½ cup	finely chopped celery
¼ cup	chopped fresh dill
¼ tsp	salt
¼ tsp	black pepper
2	tomatoes, diced
2	red bell peppers, diced
3 tbsp	chopped fresh flat-leaf parsley

Dressing:

1 tbsp	extra-virgin olive oil
1	large clove garlic, peeled and minced
½	jalapeño pepper, minced
3 tbsp	fresh lemon juice
4 cups	torn arugula or spinach leaves

1. Place the chickpeas in a food processor and pulse until finely chopped. Scrape into a large bowl. Place the shrimp in the food processor and pulse until finely chopped. Add to the chickpeas.

2. Preheat the oven to 425°F. Place the crabmeat in a fine-mesh sieve and press out any liquid. Remove any cartilage if necessary and add the crabmeat to the bowl. Add the bread crumbs, liquid egg, celery, dill, salt and pepper, and use your hands to combine until the mixture sticks together. Form the batter into 18 cakes, each about ½-inch thick. Place the cakes on a baking sheet lined with parchment paper. Bake for about 20 minutes or until golden and firm to the touch.

4. Meanwhile, combine the tomatoes, red peppers and parsley in a bowl. Set aside.

5. **Make the Dressing:** Whisk together in a small bowl the oil, garlic, jalapeño and lemon juice. Set aside.

6. Arrange the arugula on a large serving platter and top with the shrimp and crab cakes. Sprinkle with the tomato mixture and drizzle the dressing over the top just before serving.

Makes 8 to 10 servings.

QUICK FISH STEAK WITH
TOMATO CHICKPEA RELISH

GREEN-LIGHT

This recipe is so versatile, you can use fish, chicken, turkey or my favourite—lamb chops! The slight sweetness of the relish complements the peppery bite of the fish. It's perfect served with basmati rice and green beans.

Tomato Chickpea Relish:

2	large tomatoes, seeded and finely chopped
1 cup	chopped cooked chickpeas
1/3 cup	finely chopped red bell pepper
1/4 cup	finely chopped onion
1/4 cup	chopped fresh flat-leaf parsley
1/4 cup	apple cider vinegar
1 tbsp	sugar substitute
2 tsp	pickling spice
	Pinch each of salt and black pepper

Fish Steak:

1/4 cup	red wine vinegar
2 tbsp	chopped fresh thyme, or 1 tsp dried
2	cloves garlic, minced
2 tsp	Dijon mustard
1/2 tsp	black pepper
1	tuna steak (1 lb)

1. Preheat an outdoor grill or grill pan.
2. **Make the Tomato Chickpea Relish:** Stir together in a large bowl the tomatoes, chickpeas, red pepper, onion,

Complete G.I. Diet Food Guide

BEANS	RED	YELLOW	GREEN
	Baked beans with pork		Baked beans* (low fat)
	Broad		Black beans
	Refried		Black-eyed peas
			Butter beans
			Chickpeas
			Haricots
			Italian
			Mung
			Navy
			Pigeon
			Romano
			Soybeans
			Split peas

* Limit serving size (see page 63).

BEVERAGES	RED	YELLOW	GREEN
	Alcoholic drinks*	Diet soft drinks (caffeinated)	Bottled water
	Fruit drinks	Milk (1%)	Club soda
	Milk (whole or 2%)	Most unsweetened juice	Decaffeinated coffee (with skim milk, no sugar)
	Regular coffee	Red wine*	Diet soft drinks (no caffeine)
	Regular soft drinks	Vegetable juices	Herbal Teas
	Sweetened juice		Light instant chocolate
	Watermelon juice		Milk (skim)
			Soy milk (plain, low fat)
			Tea (with skim milk, no sugar)
BREADS	RED	YELLOW	GREEN
	Bagels	Crispbreads (with fibre)*	100% stone-ground whole wheat*
	Baguette/ Croissants	Pita (whole wheat)	Crispbreads (with high fibre, e.g., Wasa Fibre)*
	Cake/Cookies	Tortillas (whole wheat)	Green-light muffins (see pp. 172–75)
	Cornbread	Whole grain breads	Homemade Granola Bars (see p. 176)
	Crispbreads (regular)		Whole-grain, high-fibre breads ($2\frac{1}{2}$–3 g fibre per slice)*

* Limit serving size (see page 63).

BREADS	RED	YELLOW	GREEN
	Croutons		
	English muffins		
	Hamburger buns		
	Hot dog buns		
	Kaiser rolls		
	Melba toast		
	Muffins/Donuts		
	Pancakes/Waffles		
	Pizza		
	Stuffing		
	Tortillas		
	White bread		

CEREALS	RED	YELLOW	GREEN
	All cold cereals except those listed as yellow- or green-light	Kashi Go Lean Crunch	100% Bran
	Cereal/Granola bars	Kashi Good Friends	All-Bran
	Granola	Red River	Bran Buds
	Grits	Shredded Wheat Bran	Fibre 1
	Muesli (commercial)		Fibre First
			Homemade Muesli (see p. 87)
			Kashi Go Lean
			Oat bran
			Porridge (old-(fashioned rolled oats)

CEREAL GRAINS	RED	YELLOW	GREEN
	Couscous	Corn	Barley
	Millet		Buckwheat
	Polenta		Bulgur
	Rice (short grain, white, instant)		Quinoa
	Rice cakes		Rice (basmati, wild, brown, long grain)
			Wheat berries

CONDIMENTS/ SEASONINGS	RED	YELLOW	GREEN
	Ketchup		Capers
	Mayonnaise		Extracts (vanilla, etc.)
	Tartar sauce		Garlic
			Gravy mix (maximum 20 calories per $\frac{1}{4}$ cup serving)
			Herbs and spices
			Horseradish
			Hummus
			Mayonnaise (fat free)
			Mustard
			Salsa (no added sugar)
			Sauerkraut
			Soy sauce (low sodium)
			Teriyaki sauce
			Vinegar
			Worcestershire sauce

DAIRY	RED	YELLOW	GREEN
	Almond milk	Cheese (low fat)	Buttermilk
	Cheese	Cream cheese (light)	Cheese (fat free)
	Chocolate milk	Frozen yogurt (low fat, low sugar)	Cottage cheese (1% or fat free)
	Cottage cheese (whole or 2%)	Ice cream (low fat)	Extra low-fat cheese (e.g., Laughing Cow Light, Boursin Light)
	Cream	Milk (1%)	Fruit yogurt (nonfat with sugar substitute)
	Cream cheese	Sour cream (light)	Ice cream (low fat and
	Evaporated milk	Yogurt (low fat,) with sugar	no added sugar, e.g., Breyers Premium Fat
	Goat milk		Free, Nestlé's Legend No Added Sugar)
	Ice cream		Milk (skim)
	Milk (whole or 2%)		Soy milk (plain, low fat)
	Rice milk		Soy cheese (low fat)
	Sour Cream		
	Yogurt (whole or 2%)		

FATS AND OILS	RED	YELLOW	GREEN
	Butter	Corn oil	Almonds*
	Coconut oil	Mayonnaise (light)	Canola oil*/seed
	Hard margarine	Most nuts	Cashews*
	Lard	Natural nut butters	Flax seed
	Mayonnaise	Natural peanut butter	Hazelnuts*
	Palm oil	Peanuts	Macadamia nuts*
	Peanut butter (regular and light)	Peanut oil	Mayonnaise (fat free)

* Limit serving size (see page 63).

FATS AND OILS	RED	YELLOW	GREEN
	Salad dressings (regular)	Pecans	Olive oil*
	Tropical oils	Salad dressings (light)	Pistachios*
	Vegetable shortening	Sesame oil	Salad dressings (low fat, low sugar)
		Soft margarine (nonhydrogenated)	Soft margarine (non-hydrogenated, light)*
		Sunflower oil	Vegetable oil sprays
		Vegetable oils	
		Walnuts	

FRUITS	RED	YELLOW	GREEN
FRESH	Cantaloupe	Apricots	Apples
	Honeydew melon	Bananas	Avocado*
	Watermelon	Custard apples	Blackberries
		Kiwi	Blueberries
		Mango	Cherries
		Papaya	Cranberries
		Pineapple	Grapefruit
		Pomegranates	Grapes
			Guavas
			Lemons
			Oranges (all varieties)
			Peaches/Nectarines
			Plums
			Pears
			Raspberries
			Rhubarb
			Strawberries

* Limit serving size (see page 63).

FRUITS	RED	YELLOW	GREEN
BOTTLED, CANNED, DRIED, FROZEN	All canned fruit in syrup	Canned apricots in juice or water	Applesauce (without sugar)
	Applesauce containing sugar	Dried apricots*	Dried apples
	Most dried fruit*	Dried cranberries*	Frozen berries
		Fruit cocktail in juice	Fruit spreads (double fruit, no added sugar)
		Peaches/Pears in syrup	Mandarin oranges
			Peaches/ Pears in juice or water

JUICES**	RED	YELLOW	GREEN
	Fruit drinks	Apple (unsweetened)	
	Prune	Cranberry (unsweetened)	
	Sweetened juice	Grapefruit (unsweetened)	
	Watermelon	Orange (unsweetened)	
		Pear (unsweetened)	
		Pineapple (unsweetened)	
		Vegetable	

* For baking, it is okay to use a modest amount of dried apricots or cranberries.

* * Whenever possible, eat the fruit rather than drink its juice.

MEAT, POULTRY, FISH, EGGS AND TOFU	RED	YELLOW	GREEN
	Beef (brisket, short ribs)	Beef (sirloin steak, sirloin tip)	All fish and seafood, fresh, frozen or canned (in water)
	Bologna	Chicken/turkey leg (skinless)	Back bacon
	Breaded fish and seafood	Corned beef	Beef (top/eye round steak)
	Duck	Dried beef	Chicken breast (skinless)
	Fish canned in oil	Ground beef (lean)	Egg whites
	Goose	Lamb (fore/leg shank, centre cut loin chop)	Ground beef (extra lean)
	Ground beef (more than 10% fat)	Pork (centre loin, fresh ham, shank, sirloin, top loin)	Lean deli ham
	Hamburgers	Turkey bacon	Liquid eggs
	Hot dogs	Whole omega-3 eggs	Pastrami (turkey)
	Lamb (rack)	Tofu	Pork tenderloin
	Organ meats		Sashimi
	Pastrami (beef)		Soy cheese (low fat)
	Pâté		Tofu (low fat)
	Pork (back ribs, blade, spare ribs)		Turkey breast (skinless)
	Regular bacon		Turkey roll
	Salami		TVP (Textured Vegetable Protein)
	Sausages		Veal
	Sushi		Veggie burger
	Whole regular eggs		

PASTA*	RED	YELLOW	GREEN
	All canned pastas	Rice noodles	Capellini
	Gnocchi		Fettuccine
	Macaroni and cheese		Macaroni
			Mung bean noodles
	Noodles (canned or instant)		Penne
			Rigatoni
	Pasta filled with cheese or meat		Spaghetti/Linguine
			Vermicelli

PASTA SAUCES	RED	YELLOW	GREEN
	Alfredo	Sauces with vegetables (no added sugar)	Light sauces with vegetables (no added sugar, e.g., Healthy Choice)
	Sauces with added meat or cheese		
	Sauces with added sugar or sucrose		

SNACKS	RED	YELLOW	GREEN
	Bagels	Bananas	Almonds**
	Candy	Dark chocolate** (70% cocoa)	Applesauce (unsweetened)
	Cookies	Ice cream (low fat)	Canned peaches/pears in juice or water
	Crackers	Most nuts**	Cottage cheese (1% or fat free)
	Donuts	Popcorn (air-popped)	Extra low-fat cheese (e.g., Laughing Cow Light, Boursin Light)
	Flavoured gelatin (all varieties)		Fruit yogurt (nonfat with sugar substitute)

* Use whole-wheat or protein-enriched pastas if available.
** Limit serving size (see page 63).

SNACKS	RED	YELLOW	GREEN
	French fries		Food bars*
	Ice cream		Green-light muffins (see pp. 172–75)
	Muffins (commercial)		Hazelnuts**
	Popcorn (regular)		Homemade cookies (see pp.180–85)
	Potato chips		Homemade Granola Bars (see p. 176)
	Pretzels		Ice cream (low fat and
	Pudding		no added sugar, e.g.,
	Raisins		Breyers Premium Fat
	Rice cakes		Free, Nestlé's Legend
	Sorbet		No Added Sugar)
	Tortilla chips		Most fresh fruit
	Trail mix		Most fresh vegetables
	White bread		Pickles
			Pumpkin seeds
			Sugar-free hard candies
			Sunflower seeds
SOUPS	RED	YELLOW	GREEN
	All cream-based soups	Canned chicken noodle	Chunky bean and vegetable soups
	Canned black bean	Canned lentil	(e.g., Campbell's
	Canned green pea	Canned tomato	Healthy Request,
	Canned puréed vegetable		Healthy Choice and Too Good To Be True)
	Canned split pea		Homemade soups with green-light ingredients

* 180–225 calorie bars, e.g., Zone or Balance Bars; ½ bar per serving
** Limit serving size (see page 63).

SUGAR & SWEETENERS	RED	YELLOW	GREEN	
	Corn syrup	Fructose	Aspartame	
	Glucose		Equal	
	Honey		Splenda	
	Molasses		Stevia (note: not FDA approved)	
	Sugar (all types)		Sugar Twin	
			Sweet'N Low	

VEGETABLES	RED	YELLOW	GREEN	
	Broad beans	Artichokes	Alfalfa sprouts	Lettuce
	French fries	Beets	Asparagus	Mushrooms
	Hash browns	Corn	Beans (green/wax)	Mustard greens
				Okra
	Parsnips	Potatoes (boiled)	Bell peppers	Olives*
			Bok Choy	Onions
	Potatoes (instant)	Pumpkin	Broccoli	Peas
			Brussels sprouts	Peppers (hot)
				Pickles
	Potatoes (mashed or baked)	Squash	Cabbage (all varieties)	Potatoes (boiled new)*
			Carrots	Radicchio
	Rutabaga	Sweet potatoes	Cauliflower	Radishes
	Turnip		Celery	Rapini
		Yams	Collard greens	Snow peas
			Cucumbers	Spinach
			Eggplant	Swiss chard
			Kale	Tomatoes
			Kohlrabi	Zucchini

* Limit serving size (see page 63).

parsley, vinegar, sugar substitute, pickling spice, salt and pepper. Set aside.

3. Stir together in a large, shallow dish the vinegar, thyme, garlic, mustard and pepper. Add the fish steak and turn to coat. Let marinate for 5 minutes.
4. Place the fish steak on the greased grill over medium-high heat and grill for about 8 minutes, turning once, or until medium rare (or cook to desired doneness).
5. Cut the fish steak into 4 pieces and serve with the relish.

Makes 4 servings.

Yellow-Light Lamb Chop Option: Use 8 lean lamb chops in place of the fish steak. Increase the cooking time to 10 minutes for medium rare.

Green-Light Chicken Option: Use 4 chicken breasts, skinned, instead of the fish. Increase the cooking time to about 25 minutes.

PAN-SEARED WHITE FISH WITH MANDARIN SALSA

GREEN-LIGHT

A quick, bright citrusy salsa lends a tropical note to this hearty fish fillet. You can use tilapia, haddock or catfish for this elegant meal.

Mandarin Salsa:

2	cans (284 mL each) no-sugar-added mandarin oranges, drained
1	red bell pepper, diced
½ cup	diced cucumber
¼ cup	finely diced red onion
3 tbsp	chopped fresh cilantro
1 tbsp	rice vinegar
¼ tsp	salt
	Pinch of black pepper

Fish Fillets:

¾ cup	fresh whole wheat breadcrumbs
¼ cup	chopped fresh flat-leaf parsley
2 tbsp	wheat bran
2 tbsp	wheat germ
1 tbsp	chopped fresh tarragon, or 1 tsp dried
¼ tsp	salt
¼ tsp	black pepper
¼ cup	whole wheat flour
⅓ cup	liquid egg
4	white fish fillets (4 oz each)
4 tsp	canola oil

1. **Make the Mandarin Salsa:** Coarsely chop the mandarin slices and place them in a bowl. Add the red pepper, cucumber, onion, cilantro, rice vinegar, salt and pepper. Toss to combine.

2. **Prepare the Fish Fillets:** Prepare three large, shallow dishes. In the first combine the bread crumbs, parsley, wheat bran and germ, tarragon, salt and pepper. In the second, place the flour. In the third, place the liquid egg. Dip a fish fillet into the flour first, shaking off the excess. Then coat the fillet with liquid egg. Then dredge it evenly in the breadcrumb mixture. Repeat with the rest of the fillets. Place the prepared fillets on a plate lined with waxed paper and set aside.

3. Heat half of the oil in a large nonstick skillet over medium-high heat. Add 2 of the fillets and cook, turning once, or until golden brown, about 10 minutes. Repeat with the remaining oil and fillets. Serve topped with Mandarin Salsa.

Makes 4 servings.

Poultry

OPEN-FACED CHICKEN REUBEN SANDWICH

`GREEN-LIGHT`

The hefty Reuben sandwich has always been a big favourite with the lunch crowd at restaurants. This version is lightened up, packed with fibre and spiked with tangy spread. It's great for lunch or dinner served alongside a green salad.

Sandwich Spread:

½ cup	plain yogurt
2 tsp	balsamic vinegar
1	hard-boiled egg, finely chopped
2 tsp	minced pitted green olives
2 tsp	minced red bell pepper
½ tsp	Worcestershire sauce
4 slices	stone-ground whole wheat bread
3 cups	shredded cooked chicken (see Hint)
2 cups	shredded cabbage
1	tomato, sliced
4 slices	light-style Swiss cheese
2 tsp	nonhydrogenated soft margarine or canola oil

1. **Make the Sandwich Spread:** Whisk together in a small bowl the yogurt, vinegar, egg, olives, red pepper and Worcestershire sauce.

2. Slather each piece of bread with equal portions of the spread. Top with chicken, cabbage and tomato. Lay one slice of cheese on each sandwich.
3. Preheat the oven to 400°F.
4. Melt the margarine in a large ovenproof nonstick skillet over medium-high heat. Place the sandwiches in the skillet, in batches if necessary, and cook until the bread is toasted, about 5 minutes. Place the skillet in the oven until the cheese melts, about 5 minutes.

Makes 4 servings.

Helpful Hint: You can use leftover grilled or roasted chicken or turkey. Or you can pick up 2 cooked chicken legs at the grocery store; with skin and bones removed, you should have about 3 cups of meat.

BASMATI RICE PAELLA GREEN-LIGHT

This dish is a crowd pleaser—perfect for entertaining. Have a themed party with other Spanish foods like wilted greens or stewed chickpeas.

1 tbsp	extra-virgin olive oil
1 lb	boneless, skinless chicken thighs
1	onion, chopped
4	cloves garlic, minced
1	red bell pepper, chopped
1	green bell pepper, chopped
4 cups	chicken broth (low-fat, low-sodium)
1	can (796 mL) diced tomatoes
1 tbsp	paprika
$\frac{1}{4}$ tsp	saffron threads
1 $\frac{1}{2}$ cups	basmati rice
8 oz	green beans, trimmed
1 cup	fresh or frozen lima beans
1 cup	fresh or frozen peas
1 lb	large raw shrimp, peeled and deveined
1 lb	mussels, rinsed

1. Heat the oil in a large, shallow Dutch oven or a deep non-stick skillet over medium-high heat. Add the chicken pieces and cook on both sides until browned. Remove them to a plate.
2. Reduce the heat to medium. Add the onion, garlic and peppers and cook until the onion has softened, about 5 minutes. Add the chicken broth, tomatoes, paprika and

saffron and bring to a boil. Stir in the rice, chicken and pan juices, reduce the heat to low, and simmer uncovered, gently, for about 20 minutes.

3. Meanwhile, cut the green beans into 1-inch pieces. Gently stir the beans, lima beans and peas into the rice mixture. Stir in the shrimp and mussels, cover, and cook for about 15 minutes or until the rice is tender and the mussels are open.

Makes 6 to 8 servings.

Helpful Hint: Mussels that do not stay closed before cooking need to be discarded. Simply tap them gently on the counter to see if they will stay closed. Cooked mussels that remain closed after cooking must be discarded too.

SPINACH-STUFFED TURKEY BREAST `GREEN-LIGHT`

Veggies are great on the side, but they also add tons of flavour and nutrition when served right in your meat. Try Swiss chard instead of the spinach in this recipe for a slightly sharper flavour.

1 tsp	canola oil
½ cup	chopped green onions
1	clove garlic, minced
½	red bell pepper, finely diced
½	yellow bell pepper, finely diced
1 cup	cooked red kidney beans, mashed
1 tbsp	finely chopped fresh ginger
2 cups	chopped spinach
2 tbsp	chopped fresh mint
¼ tsp	salt
¼ tsp	black pepper
1	boneless turkey breast (about 2 lbs)

Sesame Garlic Marinade:

3 tbsp	soy sauce
2 tbsp	rice vinegar
2	cloves garlic, minced
2 tsp	sesame oil
½ tsp	Asian chili paste or Tabasco sauce

1. Heat the oil in a large nonstick skillet over medium heat. Add the green onions and garlic and cook until the green onions are beginning to soften, about 3 minutes.

Add the red and yellow peppers, beans and ginger, and cook, stirring, for 2 minutes. Add the spinach, cover, and cook, stirring occasionally, until wilted, about 5 minutes. Remove the skillet from the heat. Add the mint, salt and pepper. Let cool completely.

2. Remove the skin from the turkey and discard. Using a chef's knife, slice the turkey breast horizontally in half almost all the way through. Open the meat like a book, and using a meat mallet, pound the turkey to about ½ inch thick. Spread the spinach mixture over the turkey breast. Roll up the meat like a jelly roll, and, using kitchen string, tie the roll at 2-inch intervals. Place the tied roll in a small, shallow roasting pan.

3. **Make the Sesame Garlic Marinade:** Whisk together in a small bowl the soy sauce, rice vinegar, garlic, sesame oil and Asian chili paste. Pour the marinade over the turkey breast, turning to coat all sides. Cover with plastic wrap and refrigerate for at least 1 hour or for up to 4 hours.

4. Preheat the oven to 325°F. Roast the turkey for about 1 hour and 15 minutes or until a meat thermometer reaches 180°F. Let stand for 10 minutes before slicing into ½-inch-thick slices. Or, let the turkey cool completely and refrigerate until cold. Cut into thin slices and serve.

Makes 6 to 8 servings.

CHICKEN JAMBALAYA

GREEN-LIGHT

Jambalaya is a traditional Cajun dish in which rice is used to sop up the rich juices of the stew.

2 tsp	canola oil
2	stalks celery, chopped
2	cloves garlic, minced
1	onion, chopped
1 lb	boneless, skinless chicken, cut into ½-inch cubes
2 tsp	dried thyme
2 tsp	dried oregano
1 tsp	chili powder
¼ tsp	cayenne pepper (optional)
2 cups	chicken broth (low-fat, low-sodium)
2	green bell peppers, diced
1	can (796 mL) stewed tomatoes
1	can (540 mL) kidney beans, drained and rinsed
¾ cup	brown rice
1	bay leaf
¼ cup	chopped fresh flat-leaf parsley

1. Heat the oil in a Dutch oven over medium-high heat. Add the celery, garlic and onion and cook until the onion has softened, about 5 minutes. Add the chicken, thyme, oregano, chili powder and cayenne and cook, stirring, for 5 minutes.
2. Add the chicken broth, green peppers, tomatoes, kidney beans, rice, and bay leaf and bring to a boil. Reduce

the heat to low, cover and simmer, stirring occasionally, for about 35 minutes or until the rice is tender. Let the dish stand for 5 minutes. Remove the bay leaf and discard. Stir in the parsley before serving.

Makes 4 servings.

Turkey Option: Use boneless, skinless turkey instead of the chicken.

Seafood Option: Add 8 oz of small raw shrimp, peeled and deveined, during the last 10 minutes of cooking.

Meat

SPAGHETTI AND MEATBALLS `GREEN-LIGHT`

A home-cooked meal is a wonderful thing to come home to, and this one is a favourite of many. You can make the meatballs ahead and freeze them.

1	egg
⅓ cup	fresh whole wheat bread crumbs
¼ cup	wheat bran
¼ cup	chopped fresh flat-leaf parsley
1	clove garlic, minced
¼ tsp	salt
¼ tsp	black pepper
12 oz	lean ground turkey or chicken
2 cups	low-fat chunky vegetable pasta sauce
1 cup	cooked chickpeas
½	green bell pepper, diced
6 oz	whole wheat spaghetti

1. Preheat the oven to 350°F. Stir together in a large bowl the egg, bread crumbs, bran, parsley, garlic, salt and pepper. Work the ground turkey in with your hands until well combined. Roll the mixture into 1-inch round meatballs and place on a baking sheet lined with aluminum foil. Bake for about 12 minutes or until no longer pink inside.
2. Meanwhile, bring a large pot of salted water to a boil.

3. In a separate large saucepan cook the pasta sauce, chickpeas and green pepper over medium heat. Add the meatballs and simmer for 15 minutes.

4. Cook the pasta in the boiling water until al dente, about 10 minutes. Remove the meatballs to a small serving bowl. Drain the pasta and add it to the pasta sauce, tossing to coat well. Serve with the meatballs.

Makes 4 servings.

Make Ahead: Let meatballs cool completely and freeze in an airtight container for up to 2 months.

Helpful Hint: To make your own pasta sauce, purée 2 cans (796 mL each) plum tomatoes. Place in a saucepan over medium heat along with 1 onion, chopped, 2 cloves garlic, minced, 1 zucchini, chopped, 1 red bell pepper, chopped, 2 tsp dried oregano and ½ tsp each salt and black pepper. Bring to a boil and simmer for about 40 minutes or until thickened slightly. Keep refrigerated for up to 1 week or freeze for up to 1 month.

BAKED BEANS

GREEN-LIGHT

Normally, baked beans are packed with sugar and molasses, which add lots of calories. Our version achieves the same comforting, filling and fibre-packed dish without the sugar.

2 cups	dry navy or small white beans
8 cups	water
1	can (796 mL) diced tomatoes
4 oz	lean Black Forest ham, chopped
1	large red onion, finely chopped
1	can (156 mL) tomato paste
¼ cup	brown sugar substitute
2 tbsp	Dijon mustard
1 tbsp	Worcestershire sauce
2 tsp	Tabasco sauce
½ tsp	salt
½ tsp	black pepper

1. Rinse the beans and place them in a Dutch oven filled with water. Cover, and let soak overnight. The next day drain and rinse the beans.
2. In the same pot, add the 8 cups of water and the beans and bring to a boil. Reduce the heat, cover, and simmer, stirring occasionally, for about 1 ½ hours or until the beans are tender. Drain the beans, reserving the cooking liquid.
3. Preheat the oven to 300°F.
4. In a large bean pot or the same Dutch oven, combine

1 cup of the reserved cooking liquid, the beans, tomatoes, ham, onion, tomato paste, brown sugar substitute, mustard, Worcestershire sauce, Tabasco, salt and pepper. Cover, and bake, stirring occasionally, for 2 ½ hours. Uncover, and cook for 1 hour or until thickened.

Makes 8 servings.

Quick-Soak Option: Rinse the beans and place them in a Dutch oven filled with water. Bring to a boil and cook for 2 minutes. Cover, remove from the heat, and let sit for an hour. Then drain and continue with the recipe.

Slow-Cooker Option: Place the cooked beans with the rest of the ingredients in a slow cooker and cook on Low for 8 to 10 hours or on High for 4 to 6 hours or until tender.

SLOPPY JOES GREEN-LIGHT

Here's a meal that is great for lunch and dinner. It hits home for the whole family on a cold winter night or after a weekend hockey game. Serve it with freshly cut veggies and hummus for dipping.

1 lb	extra-lean ground beef
1	onion, chopped
4	cloves garlic, minced
1	green bell pepper, chopped
½	jalapeño pepper, minced
1	can (540 mL) red kidney beans, drained and rinsed
1	can (796 mL) diced tomatoes
¼ cup	old-fashioned rolled oats
1 tbsp	chili powder
2 tsp	Worcestershire sauce
4	whole wheat pita halves
2 cups	chopped romaine or iceberg lettuce
2	tomatoes, chopped

1. Cook the beef in a large, deep nonstick skillet or Dutch oven over medium-high heat until browned, about 8 minutes. Add the onion, garlic, green pepper, and jalapeño pepper and cook for 5 minutes. Add the beans, tomatoes, oats, chili powder and Worcestershire sauce and bring to a boil. Reduce the heat and simmer, stirring occasionally, until thickened, about 25 minutes.

2. Scoop the sloppy joe mixture into pita halves and top with lettuce and tomato.

Makes 4 to 6 servings.

Lighter Option: You can use ground turkey or chicken instead of beef.

Vegetarian Option: You can use ground meat substitute instead of the beef.

Chili Option: To serve this as a chili, simply reduce the cooking time to about 15 minutes.

STEAK FETTUCCINE

GREEN-LIGHT

A steak with a serving of pasta sounds like old-fashioned, fattening fare. Not our version. The meat is marinated with a peppery dressing and served, sliced, atop fettuccine dressed with a fresh tomato sauce. The result is light and flavourful, yet elegant enough for company.

1	top sirloin grilling steak (1 lb)
2 tbsp	Dijon mustard
2 tsp	dried Italian herb seasoning
½ tsp	black pepper
	Salt
1 tsp	extra-virgin olive oil
2	shallots, thinly sliced
2	cloves garlic, minced
1 tsp	dried oregano
½ tsp	dried basil
3	tomatoes, chopped
1	red bell pepper, thinly sliced
1	orange bell pepper, thinly sliced
½ cup	beef broth (low-fat, low-sodium)
1 cup	snow peas, trimmed
6 oz	whole wheat fettuccine or linguine

1. Preheat an outdoor grill or grill pan. Trim any fat from the steak and discard.
2. Stir together in a small bowl the mustard, Italian herb seasoning and black pepper. Spread evenly over the steak. Place the steak on the greased grill over medium-high

heat and grill for about 8 minutes, turning once, or until medium rare inside. Remove to a plate, cover, and keep warm.

3. Bring a large pot of salted water to a boil.

4. Heat the oil in a nonstick skillet over medium-high heat. Add the shallots, garlic, oregano and basil and cook until the shallots are starting to become golden, about 5 minutes. Add the tomatoes, bell peppers and broth, and bring to a boil. Reduce the heat and simmer gently until the tomatoes are starting to break down, about 5 minutes. Add the snow peas and cook until bright green, about 3 minutes. Stir in ¼ tsp salt.

5. Cook the fettuccine in the boiling salted water until al dente, about 10 minutes. Drain well and return the pasta to the pot. Toss with the sauce to coat. Place the pasta in a large serving dish. Thinly slice the steak across the grain and lay on top of the fettuccine. Serve immediately.

Makes 4 servings.

CLASSIC MEAT LASAGNA   GREEN-LIGHT

In a traditional lasagna, cheese adds a delicious creamy
layer—as well as a lot of calories. You can get that same rich
flavour with a green-light béchamel sauce.

1 lb	extra-lean ground beef or veal
1	onion, finely chopped
4	cloves garlic, minced
8 oz	mushrooms, sliced
2	zucchini, trimmed and chopped
1	each red and green bell pepper, chopped
1 tbsp	dried oregano
1/2 tsp	red pepper flakes
1/2 cup	beef broth (low-fat, low-sodium)
2	cans (796 mL each) plum tomatoes, puréed
1/4 tsp	each salt and black pepper
12	whole-wheat lasagna noodles

Béchamel Sauce:

1/4 cup	canola oil
1/2 cup	whole wheat flour
4 cups	warm skim milk
2 tbsp	grated Parmesan cheese
1/4 tsp	each salt and black pepper
	Pinch of nutmeg

1. Cook the ground beef, onion and garlic in a deep
   nonstick skillet over medium heat until browned, about 8
   minutes. Add the mushrooms, zucchini, bell peppers,

oregano and red pepper flakes, and cook, stirring occasionally, until the onion has softened, about 10 minutes. Add the broth and bring it to a boil. Let cook until all the liquid has evaporated, then add the puréed tomatoes, salt and pepper and bring to a boil again. Reduce the heat and simmer until thickened, about 30 minutes.

2. Bring a large pot of salted water to a boil.

3. **Make the Béchamel Sauce:** Heat the oil in a saucepan over medium-high heat. Add the flour and cook, stirring, for 1 minute. Slowly pour in the milk and whisk to combine. Cook, whisking gently, until the mixture thickens, about 5 minutes. Add the Parmesan cheese, salt, pepper, and nutmeg. Remove from the heat.

4. Meanwhile, cook the lasagna noodles in the boiling water until al dente, about 10 minutes. Drain, and rinse under cold water. Lay the noodles flat on damp tea towels and set aside. Preheat the oven to 350°F.

5. Ladle 1 ½ cups of the meat sauce in the bottom of a 9 x 13-inch glass baking dish. Lay 3 noodles on top of the sauce. Spread with another 1 cup of the meat sauce, then one fourth of the béchamel sauce. Repeat the layers—noodles, meat sauce, béchamel sauce—ending with béchamel sauce. Cover the dish with aluminum foil and place it on a baking sheet. Bake for 45 minutes, then uncover and bake for 15 minutes or until bubbly. Cool 10 minutes before serving.

Makes 8 servings.

Snacks

OVER-THE-TOP BRAN MUFFINS WITH PEAR

`GREEN-LIGHT`

These muffins are big and full of fibre. They are "Over-the-Top" because they rise above the top of the pan, so be sure to grease the top of your muffin pan too. The addition of fresh, chopped pear keeps these muffins moist.

1 cup	All-Bran or 100% Bran cereal
1 cup	wheat bran
1 ½ cups	plain low-fat yogurt
2 cups	whole wheat flour
½ cup	brown sugar substitute
1 tbsp	baking powder
2 tsp	baking soda
¼ tsp	salt
½ cup	skim milk
¼ cup	canola oil
1	egg
2 tsp	vanilla extract
2	pears, cored and diced

1. Combine the cereal and wheat bran in a bowl. Stir in the yogurt and let stand for 10 minutes.
2. In a separate bowl, combine the flour, brown sugar substitute, baking powder, baking soda and salt.
3. Add the milk, oil, egg and vanilla to the bran mixture

and stir to combine. Pour over the flour mixture and stir until just combined. Stir in the pear.

4. Preheat the oven to 375°F. Divide the batter among 12 greased or paper-lined muffin cups. Bake until the tops are golden and firm to the touch, about 25 minutes. Let cool on a rack for 5 minutes. Remove the muffins from the pan and let cool completely.

Makes 12 muffins.

Dried Fruit Option: Use 1 cup dried cranberries, raisins, diced apricots or dried blueberries instead of the pear.

Blueberry Option: Use 2 cups fresh blueberries instead of the pear.

Storage: Wrap each muffin individually in plastic wrap and freeze in an airtight container for up to 1 month or keep at room temperature in an airtight container for up to 3 days.

APPLE BRAN MUFFINS   GREEN-LIGHT

Ruth created this recipe several years ago when I was trying to lose weight. We'd make large batches of them and freeze them. Then, whenever I needed a snack, I'd warm one up in the microwave. They were so convenient—not to mention delicious.

	Vegetable oil cooking spray
¾ cup	All-Bran or Bran Buds cereal
1 cup	skim milk
⅔ cup	whole wheat flour
⅓ cup	sugar substitute
2 tsp	baking powder
½ tsp	baking soda
¼ tsp	salt
1 tsp	ground allspice
½ tsp	ground cloves
1 ½ cups	oat bran
⅔ cup	raisins
1	large apple, peeled and cut into ¼-inch cubes
1	omega-3 egg, lightly beaten
2 tsp	vegetable oil
½ cup	applesauce (unsweetened)

1 Preheat the oven to 350°F. Spray a 12-cup muffin tin with vegetable oil cooking spray.
2. Mix the cereal and skim milk in a bowl and let stand for a few minutes.

3. In a large bowl, mix the flour, sugar substitute, baking powder, baking soda, salt, allspice and cloves. Stir in the oat bran, raisins and apple.
4. In a small bowl, combine the egg, oil and applesauce. Stir, along with the bran mixture, into the dry ingredients.
5. Spoon the batter into the prepared muffin tin. Bake until lightly browned, about 20 minutes.

Makes 12 muffins.

HOMEMADE GRANOLA BARS   `GREEN-LIGHT`

These bars are very nutritious and really satisfy.

1 ⅓ cups	whole wheat flour
⅓ cup	sugar substitute
2 tsp	baking powder
¼ cup	All-Bran or Bran Buds cereal
1 tsp	each ground cinnamon and allspice
½ tsp	each ground ginger and salt
1 ½ cups	old-fashioned rolled oats
1 cup	finely chopped dried apricots
½ cup	shelled sunflower seeds
¾ cup	applesauce (unsweetened)
½ cup	apple juice (unsweetened)
3	omega-3 eggs
2 tsp	vegetable oil

1. Preheat the oven to 400°F. Line a shallow 8 x 12-inch baking dish with parchment paper.
2. Mix the flour, sugar substitute, baking powder, cereal, cinnamon, allspice, ginger and salt in a large bowl. Stir in the oats, apricots and sunflower seeds.
3. Mix the applesauce, apple juice, eggs and oil, and add to the flour mixture. Pour the batter into the prepared baking dish and spread it out evenly.
4. Bake until lightly browned, 15 to 20 minutes. Let cool and cut into 16 bars.

Makes 16 bars.

OATCAKES

These Scottish treats have been around for a long time. Traditionally they were made without sweetening, but over time the sweetened version appeared and people were hooked. You can try these without the sugar substitute and see which version you prefer.

2 cups	old-fashioned rolled oats
1 cup	whole wheat flour
½ cup	wheat bran
⅓ cup	sugar substitute
½ tsp	salt
½ cup	nonhydrogenated soft margarine
1	egg, lightly beaten
3 tbsp	water

1. Combine the oats, flour, bran, sugar substitute and salt in a large bowl. Use a wooden spoon to stir in the margarine until a crumbly mixture forms. Add the egg and water and stir until the dough sticks together.
2. Preheat the oven to 350°F. Divide the dough into 16 pieces. Form each piece into a ¼-inch-thick round and place on a baking sheet lined with parchment paper. Bake for 15 minutes. Turn the oatcakes over and bake on the other side until firm and golden, about 10 minutes.

Makes 16 oatcakes.

BLUEBERRY BARS

GREEN-LIGHT

This breakfast bar spinoff contains much more fibre and far fewer calories than store-bought ones. You can make them on the weekend to snack on through the week.

2 ½ cups	frozen blueberries
¼ cup	water
2 tbsp	sugar substitute
½ tsp	grated lemon zest
2 tsp	fresh lemon juice
1 tbsp	cornstarch
1 cup	old-fashioned rolled oats
¾ cup	whole wheat flour
¾ cup	wheat bran
½ cup	brown sugar substitute
¼ tsp	baking soda
½ cup	soft nonhydrogenated margarine
3 tbsp	liquid egg

1. Bring the blueberries, water, sugar substitute, lemon zest and juice, and cornstarch to a boil in a saucepan over medium heat. Cook, stirring, until thickened and bubbly, about 2 minutes. Let cool.
2. Preheat the oven to 350°F.
3. Combine the oats, flour, bran, brown sugar substitute and baking soda in a bowl. Use a wooden spoon to work in the margarine until the mixture resembles coarse crumbs. Add the liquid egg and stir until moistened. Reserve ¾ cup of the mixture for the top. Press

the remaining mixture into the bottom of an 8-inch baking pan lined with parchment paper. Spread with blueberry filling. Sprinkle with the reserved oat mixture.

4. Bake until the crust is golden and the blueberry filling is bubbly at the edges, about 30 minutes. Let cool completely before cutting into bars.

Makes 24 bars.

Storage: Place bars in an airtight container and keep refrigerated for up to 5 days or freeze for up to 2 weeks.

Desserts

OATMEAL COOKIES

GREEN-LIGHT

These soft cookies make a homey afternoon snack with a glass of milk. They are also perfect for lunch bags. Kids and adults alike are always happy to find a cookie in their brown bags.

2 cups	old-fashioned rolled oats
¾ cup	whole wheat flour
½ cup	wheat bran
½ tsp	baking soda
½ tsp	ground cinnamon
	Pinch of salt
1 cup	brown sugar substitute
½ cup	nonhydrogenated soft margarine
¼ cup	liquid egg
¼ cup	water
2 tsp	vanilla extract
½ cup	dried currants (optional)

1. Stir together in a bowl the oats, flour, bran, baking soda, cinnamon and salt. Set aside.
2. In another large bowl, beat the brown sugar substitute, margarine, liquid egg, water and vanilla until smooth. Stir the oat mixture into the margarine mixture until

combined. Add the currants, if using, and stir to combine. Preheat the oven to 375°F.

3. Drop the dough by heaping tablespoonfuls onto a baking sheet lined with parchment paper and flatten slightly. Bake until firm and golden on bottom, about 8 minutes. Repeat with the remaining dough. Let cool on a rack.

Makes about 28 cookies.

Storage: Keep in an airtight container for up to 3 days or freeze for up to 1 month.

CHEWY PEANUT BARS

`YELLOW-LIGHT`

Here's a chewy granola treat that's sure to be a hit with the whole family.

1 ½ cups	old-fashioned rolled oats
¼ cup	chopped unsalted peanuts (optional)
½ cup	wheat bran
⅓ cup	whole wheat flour
½ tsp	each baking soda and baking powder
	Pinch each of salt and ground cinnamon
⅔ cup	liquid egg
½ cup	smooth peanut butter (natural, no sugar added)
¼ cup	brown sugar substitute
2 tsp	vanilla extract

1. Combine in a large bowl the oats, peanuts (if using), wheat bran, flour, baking soda, baking powder, salt and cinnamon. Preheat the oven to 350°F.
2. In another bowl, beat the liquid egg, peanut butter, brown sugar substitute and vanilla until combined. Add the oat mixture and stir to combine. Scrape the dough into an 8-inch square baking pan lined with parchment paper. With damp hands, press down the mixture to flatten evenly. Bake until firm to the touch, about 12 minutes. Let cool and cut into bars.

Makes 12 bars.

CHOCOLATE DROP COOKIES   `GREEN-LIGHT`

These moist cookies are wonderful dunked into a glass of milk. Though beans might seem an odd addition, trust us, they keep the batter tender and sneak in some extra fibre.

½ cup	cooked white kidney beans
1 tbsp	wheat bran
¼ cup plus 2 tbsp skim milk	
⅓ cup	nonhydrogenated soft margarine
¾ cup	whole-wheat flour
½ cup	sugar substitute
⅓ cup	unsweetened cocoa powder
1	egg
2 tsp	vanilla extract
½ tsp	baking soda

1. Put the white kidney beans, wheat bran, and 2 tbsp skim milk into a food processor and purée until well blended. Set aside.
2. Put the margarine, flour, sugar substitute, bean purée, cocoa powder, the remaining skim milk, the egg, vanilla and baking soda in a bowl and beat until combined.
3. Preheat the oven to 375°F. Drop the batter by tablespoons onto a baking sheet lined with parchment paper. Bake until firm to the touch, about 10 minutes. Let cool on a rack.

Makes about 24 cookies.

CHOCOLATE ALMOND SLICES   `GREEN-LIGHT`

These are similar to biscotti in that they are baked twice.
Adults and kids love them and they keep well. You can add
¼ cup of dried cranberries or raisins for some colour and
extra flavour, if desired.

¼ cup	nonhydrogenated soft margarine
½ cup	sugar substitute
½ cup	liquid egg
4 tsp	vanilla extract
¼ tsp	almond extract (optional)
½ cup	unsweetened cocoa
½ cup	wheat bran
¼ cup	wheat germ
½ cup	whole wheat flour
2 tsp	baking powder
	Pinch of salt
½ cup	slivered almonds

1. Cream together in a large bowl the margarine and sugar
   substitute. Beat in the liquid egg, vanilla and almond
   extract, if using. Beat in the cocoa, wheat bran, wheat
   germ, half of the flour, the baking powder and salt. Stir
   in the remaining flour and knead in the almonds with
   your hands.
2. Preheat the oven to 350°F.
3. Shape the dough into 2 logs, each about 10 inches
   long, and place them on a baking sheet lined with
   parchment paper. Flatten each slightly.

4. Bake for about 20 minutes or until firm. Let the pan cool on a rack for about 15 minutes. Turn the oven down to 300°F. Use a knife to cut each log diagonally into ½-inch slices. Place the slices on a baking sheet, cut sides down. Bake, turning once, until crisp, about 15 minutes. Let cool completely before serving.

Makes about 2 dozen cookies.

Storage: Keep in a resealable plastic bag or airtight container at room temperature for up to 5 days or freeze for up to 1 month.

FRUIT AND YOGURT PARFAITS   `GREEN-LIGHT`

Enjoy these parfaits for breakfast, a snack or dessert. Use whatever fruit is seasonal—blueberries, strawberries and apples all work well.

2 cups	old-fashioned rolled oats
½ cup	wheat germ
⅓ cup	wheat bran
¼ cup	slivered almonds
¼ cup	shelled unsalted sunflower seeds
2 tbsp	sugar substitute
1 tbsp	canola oil
1 tbsp	water
2 tsp	grated orange zest
1 tsp	vanilla extract
	Pinch of salt
½ cup	raisins or dried cranberries
1	tub (750 g) nonfat, fruit-flavoured yogurt with sugar substitute
2 cups	chopped fresh fruit or berries

1. Toss together in a large bowl the oats, wheat germ and bran, almonds and sunflower seeds.
2. Preheat the oven to 300°F.
3. In a small bowl, whisk together the sugar substitute, oil, water, orange zest, vanilla and salt. Pour over the oat mixture and toss well to coat evenly. Spread the mixture onto a large baking sheet lined with parchment paper and

bake, stirring once, until golden brown, about 30 minutes. Let cool completely. Add the raisins, stirring to combine.

4. In a large glass serving bowl, layer 1 cup of the yogurt then half of the granola. Repeat once and top with the remaining yogurt. Sprinkle the fruit on top.

Makes 6 servings.

Storage: Cover and refrigerate for up to 2 days. Note that as the parfait sits, the granola softens.

Granola Storage: Keep in a resealable plastic bag or airtight container at room temperature for up to 3 days.

Yogurt Cheese Option: Use yogurt cheese (page 190) instead of yogurt.

CRUSTLESS FRUIT-TOPPED CHEESECAKE

GREEN-LIGHT

The best part of cheesecake is the rich filling, so we've eliminated the crust and focused on the middle and top layers. You can change the topping according to what fruit is in season.

1	tub (500 g) 1% cottage cheese
1	package (250 g) light cream cheese, softened
1 cup	nonfat, fruit-flavoured yogurt with sugar substitute
³/₄ cup	sugar substitute
¼ cup	cornstarch
2	egg whites
1 tbsp	vanilla extract
	Pinch of salt

Fruit Topping:

4 cups	fresh raspberries, blueberries or sliced strawberries
2 tsp	fresh lemon juice
	Sugar substitute

1. Purée the cottage cheese in a food processor until very smooth. Add the cream cheese and purée until smooth and combined. Add the yogurt, sugar substitute, cornstarch, egg whites, vanilla and salt and purée until smooth.
2. Preheat the oven to 325°F.

3. Pour the batter into a greased and parchment-lined 8- or 9-inch springform pan. Wrap the pan with aluminum foil so that the bottom and sides of the pan are covered. Place in a large roasting pan and fill the roasting pan with hot water to come halfway up the sides of the springform pan.

4. Bake until the centre is slightly jiggly when the pan is tapped, about 40 minutes. Turn the oven off and run a small knife around the edge of the pan. Let the cake stand in the cooling oven for about 30 minutes more. Remove to a rack and let cool to room temperature. Cover, and refrigerate until chilled, about 2 hours

5. **Fruit Topping:** Meanwhile, combine in a large bowl the raspberries, lemon juice and sugar substitute to taste. Cut the cheesecake into wedges and serve with the fruit topping.

Makes 8 servings.

Storage: Keep the cheesecake covered and refrigerated for up to 3 days.

ALMOND-CRUSTED PEARS   `GREEN-LIGHT`

This dessert makes an elegant ending at a dinner party. The crunchy almond crust contrasts nicely with the tender flesh of the pears.

1 cup	plain low-fat yogurt
4 tbsp	sugar substitute
½ tsp	grated orange zest (optional)
¾ cup	sliced almonds
2 tbsp	wheat germ
4	ripe Bartlett or Bosc pears, cored
2 tbsp	liquid egg
½ cup	pear nectar or juice

1. **Make the Yogurt Cheese:** Place the yogurt in a sieve lined with cheesecloth or a coffee filter. Place the sieve over a bowl. Cover with plastic wrap and refrigerate for at least 1 hour or for up to 4 hours. Discard the liquid that drains off and transfer the yogurt cheese to another bowl. Add 2 tbsp of the sugar substitute and the orange zest and stir to combine. Cover with plastic wrap and refrigerate.
2. Use your hands to crush the almonds slightly, then place them in a shallow dish. Add the wheat germ and the remaining sugar substitute and stir to combine.
3. Preheat the oven to 400°F. Fill the pears loosely with the almond mixture. Brush each pear with a light coating of liquid egg, then roll and press the pears into the almond mixture. Place the coated pears in an 8-inch

square baking dish, standing upright. Pour the pear nectar in the bottom of the dish and sprinkle any remaining almond mixture into the pan. Cover the dish lightly with aluminum foil and bake until a knife inserts easily into the pears, about 30 minutes. Remove the foil and bake until the crust is golden and the juices have thickened, about 10 minutes. Let cool slightly. Serve the pears with some of the juice from the pan and the yogurt cheese.

Makes 4 servings.

FRUIT-FILLED PAVLOVA

GREEN-LIGHT

Pavlovas are meringues filled with whipped cream and fruit. We use tofu and yogurt cheese in place of the whipped cream—delicious!

8	egg whites
½ tsp	cream of tartar
	Pinch of salt
¾ cup	sugar substitute
2 tbsp	cornstarch
2 tsp	vanilla extract

Fruit Filling:

1	package (300 g) soft silken tofu, drained
1 cup	yogurt cheese (page 190)
¼ cup	sugar substitute
½ tsp	grated orange zest
4 cups	mixed fruit (such as fresh berries and orange and peach wedges)
2 tbsp	chopped fresh mint

1. Put the egg whites in a large bowl and beat with an electric mixer until frothy. Add the cream of tartar and salt and beat until soft peaks form. Gradually add the sugar substitute and beat until the peaks become stiff. Beat in the cornstarch and vanilla to combine.

2. Preheat the oven to 275°F. Spread the mixture into an 8-inch round on a baking sheet lined with parchment paper. Mound the edges slightly higher than the centre

to form a shell. Bake until lightly golden, about 40 minutes. Turn off the oven and let the meringue rest in the oven for 1 hour. Remove to a large serving platter.

3. **Make the Fruit Filling:** Meanwhile, combine in a large bowl the tofu, yogurt cheese, sugar substitute and orange zest. Scrape into the meringue shell and top with the fruit mixture. Sprinkle with mint before serving.

Makes 8 to 10 servings.

Storage: The pavlova shell can be made up to 4 hours ahead. Fill it with the fruit filling no more than 1 hour before serving.

FROZEN BLUEBERRY TREAT GREEN-LIGHT

This tangy, refreshing yogurt treat tastes like a blueberry sorbet. You can make this in an ice cream machine if you have one.

½ cup	water
½ cup	sugar substitute
3 cups	fresh blueberries
1 cup	low-fat plain yogurt

1. Bring the water and sugar substitute to a boil in a saucepan over medium heat. Remove from the heat and let cool completely.
2. Meanwhile, purée the blueberries in a food processor or blender. Add the yogurt and pulse to combine. Add the sugar substitute–water mixture and pulse to combine. Pour into an 8- or 9-inch metal cake pan and freeze until firm, about 2 hours. Cut into chunks and, working in batches, place the frozen chunks in the food processor. Purée until smooth, scrape into an airtight container, and freeze until firm.
3. Before serving, place the frozen treat in the refrigerator for 15 minutes to soften slightly.

Makes about 3 cups.

Storage: Keep tightly covered in the freezer for up to 1 week.

A Sample One-Week Green-Light Menu Plan

Monday:

Breakfast	Oatmeal (page 87)
	Tea or decaffeinated coffee
Snack	Apple Bran Muffin (page 174)
	Glass of skim milk
Lunch	Niçoise Salad (page 130)
	1 slice whole wheat bread
Snack	1% cottage cheese with orange sections and a few almonds
Dinner	Classic Meat Lasagna (page 170)
	Green salad
	Frozen Blueberry Treat (page 194)
Snack	Homemade Granola Bar (page 176)
	Glass of skim milk

Tuesday:

Breakfast	Homemade Muesli (page 87)
	Orange
	Tea or decaffeinated coffee
Snack	2 Chocolate Almond Slices (page 184)
	Pear slices
	Glass of skim milk
Lunch	Cauliflower and Chickpea Soup (page 124)
	1 slice whole wheat bread with 4 oz turkey breast, mustard, cucumber, tomato and lettuce

Snack	Laughing Cow Light cheese with celery, carrots and cherry tomatoes
Dinner	Chicken Jambalaya (page 160)
	Basmati rice
	Green salad
	Berries and nonfat yogurt
Snack	2 Oatmeal Cookies (page 180)
	Glass of skim milk

Wednesday:

Breakfast	On-the-Run Breakfast (page 88)
	Tea or decaffeinated coffee
Snack	Apple Bran Muffin (page 174)
	Glass of skim milk
Lunch	Waldorf Chicken and Rice Salad (page 94)
	Grapes
Snack	Homemade Granola Bar (page 176)
	Glass of skim milk
Dinner	Sloppy Joes (page 166)
	Hummus with cucumber, broccoli and bell pepper slices
	2 Oatmeal Cookies (page 180)
Snack	2 Chocolate Almond Slices (page 184)
	Glass of skim milk

Thursday:

Breakfast	Oatmeal (page 87)
	Tea or decaffeinated coffee

Snack	Over-the-Top Bran Muffin with Pear (page 172)
	Glass of skim milk
Lunch	Shrimp Caesar Salad (page 134)
	Canned peaches in juice
Snack	Laughing Cow Light cheese with 2 Wasa Fibre Crispbreads
Dinner	Asian Stir-fry (page 98)
	Basmati rice
	Fruit and Yogurt Parfait (page 186)
Snack	2 Blueberry Bars (page 178)
	Glass of skim milk

Friday:

Breakfast	Homemade Muesli (page 87)
	Orange
	Tea or decaffeinated coffee
Snack	2 Chocolate Almond Slices (page 184)
	Pear slices
	Glass of skim milk
Lunch	Mixed Bean Salad (page 92)
	Grapes
Snack	1% cottage cheese with fruit and almonds
Dinner	Pan-Seared White Fish with Mandarin Salsa (page 152)
	Boiled new potatoes
	Green beans
	Green salad
	½ cup low-fat, no-added-sugar ice cream

Snack	Over-the-Top Bran Muffin with Pear (page 172) Glass of skim milk

Saturday:

Breakfast	Mexican Omelette (page 89–92) Grapefruit slices Tea or decaffeinated coffee
Snack	Nonfat fruit yogurt sprinkled with Bran Buds
Lunch	Open-Faced Chicken Reuben Sandwich (page 154) Small green salad Glass of skim milk
Snack	2 Blueberry Bars (page 178) Glass of skim milk
Dinner	Steak Fettuccine (page 168) Green salad Fruit-filled Pavlova (page 192)
Snack	2 Oatmeal Cookies (page 180) Glass of skim milk

Sunday:

Breakfast	Green Eggs and Ham (page 120) Tea or decaffeinated coffee
Snack	Laughing Cow Light cheese with 2 Wasa Fibre Crispbreads
Lunch	Bean and Onion Pizza (page 138) Small green salad

	Pear
	Glass of skim milk
Snack	Hummus with cucumber and baby carrots
Dinner	Spinach-Stuffed Turkey Breast (page 158)
	Boiled new potatoes
	Broccoli
	Green salad
	Almond-Crusted Pears (page 190)
Snack	Homemade Granola Bar (page 176)
	Glass of skim milk

More delicious recipes can be found in my second book *Living the G.I. Diet.*

Dear Rick,

I have been on the G.I. diet since January and have lost 28 pounds. I feel great about myself, and am very much looking forward to being able to go for a swim this summer without being self-conscious about the way I look . . . Sincerely, this diet is one of the best things that has happened in my life and I am confident that I will never go back to eating the way I used to . . . I never thought I'd love veggies and fruit like I do now. All you have to do is give it a chance, and get into the mindset of sticking to it. The mirror is no longer my enemy!

Tim

CHAPTER NINE

Exercise

Conventional wisdom has it that exercise is an essential component of a weight loss program. Recent research findings strongly indicate that this is, in fact, *not* the case. Though any increase in an individual's level of activity is bound to burn up more calories, the net impact over the relatively short weight-loss period (typically twelve to twenty-four weeks) is small. To lose just one pound of fat, for example, a 160-pound person would have to walk briskly (4 miles per hour) for 42 miles! Over the long haul, however, to maintain your new weight, exercise is an important contributor. If you were to walk briskly for half an hour a day, seven days per week, you would burn up calories equalling twenty pounds of fat per year. This means that in Phase I, exercise is not essential to your weight-loss program, but it is an important consideration in Phase II, where you maintain your new weight.

Exercise has been an important part of my life since the age of thirty-eight, when I was humbled by my seven-year-old son. He challenged me to a run around the block—and he won soundly. I recognize that exercise is a subject many people don't want to hear about. Nevertheless, before you skip it totally, read the box below. If you still aren't convinced you should read on, then this chapter is not for you.

REGULAR EXERCISE WILL:
1. assist in weight maintenance;
2. dramatically reduce your risk of heart disease, stroke, diabetes and osteoporosis;
3. improve your mental well-being and boost your self-esteem;
4. help you to sleep better.

For those couch potatoes who have been driven by curiosity to read this far, stay with us and see if the following objections to regular exercise sound like your own: "It's painful," "It's boring," "I don't have the time." We are going to address all three complaints head-on.

Firstly, let's look at the pain or discomfort excuse. This probably comes from an experience where you've tried to do too much too soon. The world's basements are full of exercise equipment purchased in a moment of excessive enthusiasm—probably coupled with some New Year's resolutions. A few weeks later, aching muscles, a sore bottom and burning lungs have relegated that exercise bike or other exotic machine to the deep, dark storeroom where we put things that "may be useful later." Sound familiar?

To avoid pain, you must start small and work yourself up. Ten years ago I was an active jogger, running twenty-five to thirty miles a week. Unfortunately, I developed a back disc problem (totally unrelated to jogging) and it was nine years before I ventured out again. Though I kept reasonably trim during that nine-year period, I couldn't believe the problems that my re-entry to jogging created. Day One saw me enthusiastically bounding out the door in my beautiful new running shoes. Half a mile later I stopped in a wheezing heap, lungs burning, knees aching, calf muscles in spasm. You're probably thinking "serves him right," confirming for yourself that exercise is a painful option.

The reason I'm relating this story is that I had to learn the hard way. Jogging is a wonderful exercise, but it places a high demand on your body, particularly if you're over forty. Since I fell into that age category, I had to find an alternative exercise that required less physical effort and was more in tune with the realities of my aging body. I decided to start walking. Nearly everyone can walk, and if you start small and work yourself up, it is pain free (see page 208).

The second objection to exercise is boredom. I am very sympathetic to this one. While some exercises like jogging, walking and bicycling are, by their outdoor nature, rarely boring—unless people, and what they do and where they live, are of no interest to you—Canadian winters can be a disincentive. The nine years I spent working out on my exercise bike and ski machine in the basement were more of a challenge. Granted, this wasn't my only option. Many people use fitness clubs for both the motivation

("I've paid my fee, so I'd better use it") as well as the social interaction and mutual encouragement. One or two of the well-heeled have personal trainers, but this is an unrealistic option for most of us.

Instead, I chose the basement, as there was no fitness facility nearby. My solution to the inherent boredom came via an ancient TV abandoned by the children as they left the nest, and an early "replay only" VCR. I recorded those shows and films that ran between midnight and six a.m. on the family VCR, and they provided my entertainment. I pedalled and skied my way through James Bond movies, build-your-own-cottage shows and Jacques Cousteau undersea documentaries. There was never a boring moment. In fact I sometimes became so engrossed in the shows that I exercised far beyond my scheduled time allocation. Indoors, a little ingenuity (which could be as simple as putting on a Walkman), can help make workouts more interesting.

The last objection is lack of time. There are 336 thirty-minute blocks of time each week. Take 2 percent, or seven, of these blocks and use one each day. This can hardly be an unreasonable allocation of your time, especially when you consider the benefits: a slimmer, fitter, healthier you! Thirty minutes a day should be your target, though I know that many of you will want to increase this allocation once you feel the remarkable improvements that such a modest time commitment can bring.

As far as what time of day you should exercise is concerned, there are two clear camps: those who are at their best first thing in the morning and those who warm up during the day to hit their peak in the evening. I strongly suggest you align your exercise activity with whichever camp you fall into. In our household I'm the morning person, who cannot imagine exercising at the end of the day as my watchspring winds down. My wife, conversely, dreads the mornings but is a going concern by the time we get home in the evening. Needless to say, we don't exercise together. So choose your best time—either bounding out of bed to greet the dawn or exercising away accumulated tensions at the end of the day. Either way, exercise will be an enjoyable component of your daily routine.

Many people find that as their level of fitness increases, they sleep better and wake up feeling more refreshed, taking less time to drag themselves from bed. This in itself frees up more time for exercise, resulting in even less of a draw upon your day.

When referring to "exercise," we're talking about aerobic, or cardio, exercise, which boosts the heart rate and causes you to breathe harder. But before we look at exercise options and getting started, let's talk further about why we're doing this.

Weight Loss and Maintenance

One thing we need to get straight right off: exercise is *not* a substitute for dieting. Dieting will have a far greater impact on weight loss than exercise. What brought home this point to me was the annual rowing race between Oxford and Cambridge Universities on the river Thames. Rowing, along with water polo, is rated as the toughest physical endurance test for the body, and the race is over four miles long. It amazed me to find out that each rower burns the calorie equivalent of only one bar of chocolate during the race! Obviously an enormous expenditure of energy is needed to offset our poor dietary habits. But exercise is an essential complement to diet. Together, the two will give you optimum weight loss and, even more importantly, maintain your new healthy weight.

Exercise works in exactly the same way as diet to reduce or control weight. The more energy (calories) you expend than you take in, the more your body will use up your energy reserve (fat) to make up the shortfall. Exercise burns calories. In fact, every action you perform uses calories. So, climbing the stairs instead of taking the elevator to your office, getting off the bus a stop or two early, or parking as far away as possible from the mall or supermarket entrance will require extra activity over your normal routine and thereby consume extra calories. As we noted earlier, if you were to walk briskly for half an hour a day, you would lose twenty pounds a year automatically. How come? Well, a brisk half-hour walk consumes approximately 200 extra calories. Multiply that by 365 days and you get 72,000 calories, or 20 pounds (1 pound = 3,600 calories).

Note: the thirty-minute (2.5-kilometre) walk that burns 200 calories is based on a 150-pound person. Heavier people will burn more calories in thirty minutes, and lighter people will burn fewer. A 200-pound person will burn 220 calories, a 130-pound person 175 calories. And the more briskly you walk, the more calories you will consume.

Exercise has two further benefits on weight loss and control. First, exercise increases your metabolism—the rate at which you burn up calories—*even after you've finished exercising.* In other words, the benefits stay with you all day. Exercise in the morning is particularly beneficial as it sets the pace for your metabolism for the day.

A second bonus is that exercise builds muscle mass. Starting at the age of twenty-five, the body loses 1.5 percent of its muscle mass each year. This muscle turns to fat. Once men reach 60 years and women 40, the muscle loss accelerates. High-protein diets can further accelerate that loss. By exercising muscles on a regular basis, the loss can be minimized or reversed. And why is that important? Because muscles burn a lot more energy than does fat, the larger your muscles, the more energy (calories) they use. When you're at rest, or even asleep in bed, your muscles are using energy. So keeping or building muscle mass really helps you to burn calories and lose weight.

Though regular exercise will help minimize muscle loss, it is resistance exercises that actually build muscle mass. Resistance exercises are those where weights, elastic bands or hydraulics are used for muscles to pull or push against. Most of you are probably cringing at the thought of sweating body builders doing endless painful workouts with massive barbells and other daunting equipment. As we will show a little later, though, it does not have to be like that. A few simple exercises will do wonders to tone and restore those flabby muscles.

We will deal with the other health benefits of exercise in chapter 10 when we look at the impact of weight on your health, in particular on heart disease and stroke, which accounts in North America for four deaths out of every ten.

Getting Started

Now that you're convinced exercise is for you, how do you go about getting started?

1. Select an exercise that suits you. The fastest way to abandon an exercise program is to do something you don't enjoy. It is best to select an exercise that uses the largest muscle groups, that is, the legs, abdominals and lower back. These burn more calories because of their sheer size. Walking, jogging and biking are excellent choices.

2. Get support from family and friends. If possible, find a like-minded buddy so you have support.

3. Set goals and keep a record. A clippable exercise log (see page 241) is included to help keep you on track. Put it on the fridge or in the bathroom.

4. Check with your doctor to ensure that he/she supports your plan.

Now let's review your options.

Outdoor Activities

Walking

This is by far the simplest and, for most people, the easiest exercise program to start and maintain. Thirty minutes a day, seven days a week, should be your target. If you add an hour-long walk on the weekend, you can take a day off during the week. As mentioned before, we're talking about brisk walking—not speed walking or ambling. It must increase your heart and breathing rate, but never exercise to the point where you cannot find the breath to converse with a partner.

You don't need any special clothing or equipment except a pair of comfortable cushioned shoes or sneakers. And walking is rarely boring since you can keep changing routes and watch the world go by as you exercise. Walk with a friend for company and mutual support, or go solo and commune with nature and your own thoughts. I do my best thinking of the day on my morning walk. This is not surprising when you realize how much extra oxygen-fresh blood is pumping through your brain.

A great idea is to incorporate your walking into your daily commute to work. I get off the bus three stops early on my way to and from work. Those three stops are equal to about 2.5 kilometres, so I'm walking about 5 kilometres per day! If you drive to work, try parking your car about 2.5 kilometres away and walk to your job. You may even find cheaper parking farther out.

Jogging

This exercise is similar to walking, but more care is needed with footwear to protect joints from damage. The advantage of jogging over walking is that it approximately doubles the number of calories burned in the same period of time—400 calories for jogging versus 200 for brisk walking over a thirty-minute period. While walking, try jogging for a few yards and see if this is for you. It will get your heart rate up, which is great for heart health. The heart is basically a muscle, and like all muscles it thrives on being exercised—in general, the more the better. If jogging is for you, then this could arguably be the simplest and most effective method of exercise, as it uses personal time efficiently, can be done any time, anywhere, and is inexpensive.

Hiking

Another version of walking is cross-country hiking. Because this usually involves varying terrain, especially hills and valleys, you use up more calories—about 50 percent more than for brisk walking. The reason is that, going uphill, you use considerably more energy as your body literally has to lift its own weight from the bottom to the top. You try hauling 150 to 200 pounds up a hill and you'll get some idea of the extra effort your body has to make. Hiking is a great deal of fun, too, especially on weekends when you can get out of town. It also provides a change of pace from your regular walking or jogging routine.

Bicycling

Like walking, jogging and hiking, bicycling is a fun way to burn up those calories, and it is almost as effective as jogging. Again, other than the cost of the bike, it's inexpensive and can be done almost anywhere and any time. It can also be done indoors during winter months with a stationary bike.

Bicycling offers another good change of pace from your regular routine. I find it gives me a chance to visit all sorts of communities outside my normal walking range.

Other Outdoor Activities

Rollerblading, ice skating, skiing (especially cross-country), snowshoeing and swimming (in a lake or pool) are good alternatives to or changes of pace from any of the above activities. They are similar to biking in terms of energy consumption.

Sports

Though most sports are terrific calorie burners, they usually cannot be part of a regular routine. Most require other people, equipment and facilities, all of which mitigate against a continuing, regular exercise program. But again, they can be an excellent top-up or boost to your regular program. Popular sports such as golf (no golf cart, please), tennis, basketball and softball are excellent adjuncts to a basic exercise program. But they are not a substitute for a five-to-seven-days-a-week regular schedule.

Indoor Activities

Many of you will be muttering by now about how this would all sound fine if we lived in California, but get real, this is Canada; you can't do many of these activities for half the year. Though this is true in general, if you are properly attired the walking/jogging season can be extended to cover most of the year except for those days when no one wants to go outside.

The alternative is either a home gym or a fitness club. The latter is an easy option these days in most larger communities. Clubs offer not only a wide range of sophisticated equipment, but also mutual support from friends and expert advice from staff.

If a fitness club isn't convenient or those Lycra-clad young things make you uncomfortable, the simple alternative is to exercise at home. The best and least expensive equipment is a stationary exercise bike. The latest models work on magnetic resistance rather than the old friction strap around the flywheel. This gives a smoother action with better tension adjustment. Most important, they are quiet, which is crucial if you want to be able to listen to music or watch TV. (The alternative is to turn up the volume until the neighbours complain, or use a headset.)

You can easily pay into the thousands for a bike with all the fancy trimmings, one that is designed for use in a fitness club, but in reality the $250 to $350 machine will work fine. Just be sure it has smooth, adjustable tension and proper seat height, then plug in that late-night movie or your favourite soap and get pedalling. You'll be amazed how quickly the minutes fly by. I've frequently gone way over my scheduled time as I've become immersed in the screen action! Twenty minutes on the bike will give you the same calorie consumption as thirty minutes of brisk walking.

If biking is not for you, try a treadmill. These can be expensive, and beware the lower-end models that cannot take the pounding. Expect to pay about $700 to $1,000, and ensure that the incline of the track can be raised and lowered for a better workout.

Both bikes and treadmills can simulate outdoor walking, jogging, hiking or biking in the comfort of your own home. I use both of these machines but have added a cross-country ski machine, which has the advantage of working the upper body as well. Ski machines are generally less expensive than treadmills but cost more than stationary bikes. They also burn a considerably higher number of

---

Note: Most authorities support the notion that any extra activity is better than none at all. We have no argument with that, but experience shows that if people start substituting washing the car or throwing the ball for the dog as alternatives to a regular brisk exercise program, then the program does not work. By all means garden, wash the windows or whatever else you like, but please do not fool yourself into thinking that this will have a significant impact on your weight loss or maintenance program.

calories (similar to jogging) because they use arms and shoulders as well as legs—almost the perfect all-body workout machine.

There are several other more specialized options, such as stair step or rowing machines, but they are not for everyone. They are also quite expensive, so make sure you try them out first at a fitness club or with a co-operative retailer.

Resistance Training

It's now time to pay some attention to rebuilding your muscle mass. Remember that after age forty, you will lose between four and six pounds of muscle every decade. That's four to six pounds of calorie-consuming muscle. Muscles burn up energy even when idle. Let me illustrate this point. As a student I pumped gas during one of my vacations. One day a pre-war Bentley drove in and the owner asked me to fill her right to the top. He left the car running and went to the washroom. The car was filled through a large pipe that stuck about eighteen inches out of the gas tank. I was not able to fill the tank to the top of the pipe because the level kept dropping with every beat of the huge twelve-cylinder engine. I finally had to ask the owner to switch off the engine so I could finally top it up! The lesson is that, like the Bentley, bigger muscles consume more energy than smaller muscles, even when idling.

Resistance training equipment can range from the complex and expensive to the simple and inexpensive. Home gyms are a popular option for a few hundred dollars and up. For most people, however, there are much simpler methods—free weights or (my own preference) rubber bands. Dynaband and Thera-Band are two popular choices. The latter I find particularly useful as it comes in varying thicknesses, offering increasing levels of resistance as you regain and build your muscle strength.

The resistance exercises should add to your other regular exercise regimen, not replace it. Muscle-building exercise is strictly complementary to regular get-your-body-moving exercise. Using both types of exercise together will work far better than either one alone. And resistance exercises are best done every other day, leaving time for your muscles to recuperate.

For further information on resistance training, there is an excellent book titled *Strength Training Past 50* by Wayne Westcott and Thomas Baechle. Though geared to the 50-plus age group, it is useful for anyone.

Stretching

It is important to stretch at the end of your exercise program for a couple of reasons. For one, it's calming, helping you to "come down" from the intensity of your workout, and for another, it lengthens your muscles after they've been shortened and tightened while exercising. The ideal time to stretch is when the body is warmed up, either following a workout or perhaps even in the shower.

Stretching becomes even more critical as we get older. Lack of flexibility is often the reason why seniors fall or trip. Women who've made a habit of wearing high heels usually have shortened calf muscles by the time they reach their senior years and tend to shuffle as a result. That's why women trip more frequently than men and often suffer devastating hip fractures.

Staying flexible is not difficult and you can easily increase your flexibility by 100 percent in a matter of weeks. There is a wide range of books and brochures readily available on stretching exercises.

TO SUM UP:
1. A regular exercise program will accelerate weight loss and help you maintain a desired weight. It will also improve your health (especially heart health), make you feel good and allow you to sleep better. It will be the best thirty-minute-a-day investment you'll ever make.
2. Choose an activity that suits your personality and your schedule.
3. Stick to it. Make it part of your life at least five days a week—preferably every day.

CHAPTER TEN

Health

Food impacts our health in two ways. First, your choice of foods and the quantity you consume will be key determinants in how much you weigh. And the connection between being overweight and being at increased risk for diseases such as heart disease, stroke and diabetes is well-established.

Second, the types of protein, fat and carbohydrates we consume can determine your risk level for heart disease, stroke, diabetes, prostate and colon cancers and Alzheimer's. Making the right choices has been the principal theme of *The G.I.Diet*. In this chapter we will examine the role of diet in preventing diseases.

Foods are, in effect, drugs. They have a powerful influence on our health, well-being and emotional state. We take in food four or five times a day, usually with more thought for taste than for nutritional value. It would be incomprehensible to take drugs on the same basis.

The right foods can help you maintain your health, extend your lifespan, give you more energy, and make you feel good and sleep better. Couple that with exercise and you are doing all you can to keep healthy, fit and alert. The rest is a matter of genes and luck.

We'll now examine the role of diet and exercise in preventing diseases.

Heart Disease and Stroke

Given that I was the president of the Heart and Stroke Foundation of Ontario for fifteen years, it is hardly surprising that I'm starting with these diseases. However, there is a more important reason: heart disease and stroke cause 40 percent of North American deaths. Remarkably, this is evidence of progress. When I first joined the Foundation, the figure was close to 50 percent.

This is a good news, bad news story. The good news is that advances in surgery, drug therapies and emergency services have saved many lives. The bad news is that twice as many deaths could have been averted if only we had reduced our weight, exercised regularly and quit smoking. Though the smoking rate for adults has dropped sharply (unfortunately, we cannot say the same for teens), we are eating more and exercising less, leading inevitably to a more obese and unhealthy population. It's been calculated that if we led even a moderate lifestyle, we could halve the carnage from these diseases. Though heart disease, like most cancers, is primarily a disease of old age, nearly half of those who suffer heart attacks are under the age of sixty-five.

A familiar refrain that I have heard many times is, "Why worry? If I have a heart attack, today's medicine will save me." It might well save you from immediate death, but what most people do not realize is that the heart is permanently damaged after an attack. The heart cannot repair itself because its cells do not reproduce. (Ever wonder why you cannot get cancer of the heart? That's the reason.) After the damage sustained during a heart attack, the heart has to work harder to compensate—but it never can. It slowly degenerates under this stress, and patients finally "drown" as blood circulation fails and the lungs fill with liquid. Congestive heart failure is a dreadful way to die, so make sure you do everything you can to avoid having a heart attack in the first place.

With regard to diet, the simple fact is that the fatter you are, the more likely it is you will suffer a heart attack or stroke. The two key factors that link heart disease and stroke to diet are cholesterol and hypertension (high blood pressure). I promised at the beginning of this book that I was not going to dwell on the complexities of the science of nutrition; it's the outcome of this science that's important. However, a little science is helpful to understand the role and importance of both hypertension and cholesterol.

Hypertension, or high blood pressure, is the harbinger of both heart disease and stroke. High blood pressure puts more stress on the arterial system and causes it to age and deteriorate more rapidly, ultimately leading to arterial damage, blood clots, and heart attack or stroke. Excess weight has a major bearing on high blood pressure. A recent Canadian study found that obese adults, aged eighteen to fifty-five, had a five to thirteen times greater risk of hypertension. A further study demonstrated that a lower fat diet coupled with a major increase in fruits and vegetables (eight to ten servings a day) lowered blood pressure. The moral: lose weight and eat more fruits and vegetables to help reduce your blood pressure levels. In other words, adopt the G.I. Diet.

Cholesterol is essential to your body's metabolism. However, high cholesterol is a problem as it's the key ingredient in the plaque that can build up in your arteries, eventually cutting off the blood supply to your heart (causing heart attack) or your brain (leading to stroke). To make things more complicated, there are two forms of cholesterol: HDL (good) cholesterol and LDL (bad) cholesterol. The idea is to boost the HDL level while depressing the LDL level. (Remember it this way: HDL is Heart's Delight Level and LDL is Leads to Death Level.)

The villain in raising LDL levels is saturated fat, which is usually solid at room temperature and is found primarily in meat and whole milk and food products. Conversely, polyunsaturated and monounsaturated fats not only lower LDL levels but actually boost HDL. The moral: make sure some fat is included in your diet, but make sure it's the right fat. (Refer to chapter 1 for the complete rundown on fat.)

Diabetes

Diabetes is the kissing cousin of heart disease in that more people die from heart complications arising from diabetes than from diabetes alone. And diabetes rates are skyrocketing: they are expected to double in the next ten years.

The principal causes of the most common form of diabetes, Type 2, are obesity and lack of exercise, and the current epidemic is strongly correlated to the obesity trend. The most dramatic illustration of this link appears in Canada's Native population, where in some communities diabetes affects nearly half the adult population. Before the Europeans colonized North America, the Native peoples lived in a state of feast or famine. When there was an abundance of food, plant or animal, it was stored in the body as fat. In lean times, such as winter, the body depleted these fat supplies. As a result their bodies developed a "thrift gene," with those who stored and utilized their food most effectively being the survivors—a classic Darwinian exercise in survival of the fittest. When you take away the need to hunt or to harvest food—that is, the need to exercise—and replace it with a trip to the supermarket whenever food is required, the result is inevitable: a massive increase in obesity and, with it, diabetes.

Foods with a low G.I., which release sugar more slowly into the bloodstream, appear to play a major role in helping diabetics control their disease. Thus the G.I. Diet provides an opportunity both to lose weight and to assist in the management of the disease. In their magazine *Dialogue*, the Canadian Diabetes Association selected the G.I. Diet as their diet of choice. Because protein and fat have an impact on food's G.I. ratings, diabetics should be particularly careful about eating the right balance of green-light proteins, carbohydrates and fats at every meal and snack. Prevention, however, is far preferable; so get right into your G.I. Diet program and get those pounds off.

Cancer

There is increasing research evidence that diets high in saturated fat are linked to certain cancers, particularly prostate and colorectal cancer. A recent global report by the American Institute for Cancer Research concluded that 30 to 40 percent of cancers are directly linked to dietary choices. Its key recommendation is that individuals should choose a diet that includes a variety of vegetables, fruit and grains and is low in saturated fat—the G.I. Diet in a nutshell.

Alzheimer's

As with cancer, there is increasing evidence linking certain dementias, particularly Alzheimer's, with fat intake. A recent U.S. study showed a 40 percent increase in Alzheimer's disease for those who ate a diet high in saturated fat.

Abdominal Fat and Health

The most alarming medical news about fat is that it is not, as previously thought, a passive accumulator of energy reserves and extra baggage. Rather it is an active, living part of your body. Once it has formed sufficient mass, it behaves like any other organ such as the liver, heart or kidney, except that it pumps out a dangerous combination of free fatty acids and proteins. This causes out-of-control cell proliferation, which is directly associated with the growth of malignant cancer tumours. It also creates inflammation, which is linked to atherosclerosis, the principal cause of heart disease and stroke. And if that weren't bad enough, fat tissues also increase insulin resistance, leading to Type 2 diabetes.

The fact is that abdominal fat has many of the characteristics of a huge tumour—and that thought may help encourage any fence-sitters out there to start doing something about their weight.

CHAPTER ELEVEN

Supplements

As a young advertising account executive in the United Kingdom, I was briefed by a nutritionist on vitamin supplements, which Miles Labs was planning to introduce into England. The nutritionist was skeptical about the readiness of the British for these American-style multivitamin therapies and whether in fact we even needed them. Her comment—"our sewers contain the richest concentration of vitamins in the country"—still resounds in my head whenever the question of vitamins and other food supplements comes up.

There is a great deal of truth in what she said. Most of us get at least the minimum recommended levels of most vitamins and minerals from our diet. There is increasing evidence, however, that the usual RDA (Recommended Daily Allowance) may be insufficient in certain specific instances. This is a dynamic area of nutrition research and very susceptible to change as new data pours in on a daily basis. Based on our present knowledge, here are some guidelines that may be helpful.

Vitamin B

There is growing evidence that vitamin B, or more specifically B6, B12 and folic acid, are key ingredients in combatting a chemical called homocysteine, which attacks your arteries. This substance is triggered by digesting animal protein, which again suggests that high-protein diets can be dangerous to your health.

Because excessive doses of some B vitamins can be dangerous, the levels in most one-a-day multivitamins (20 mcg B12, 2 mg B6, 400 mcg folic acid) are quite sufficient as a top-up to any possible deficiencies in your diet.

Vitamin C

This is certainly the most popular vitamin sold, mainly because of its association with cold prevention and reduction. Though there is little evidence to support that traditional claim, we do know that vitamin C is critical to muscles, ligaments and joints.

While the G.I. Diet, with its emphasis on fresh fruit and vegetables, will certainly cover your basic vitamin C requirements, a top-up through a one-a-day multivitamin may help.

Vitamin D

This is the true sunshine vitamin, and not vitamin C as the Florida ads suggest. Though vitamin D is prevalent in milk and fatty fish, our body can only produce vitamin D itself when exposed to sunshine. For Canadians sunshine is a scarce commodity in winter, and since we should be lathered in sunscreen during our brief summer we are unable to capitalize on this vitamin self-generation.

Vitamin D is important because it facilitates the processing of calcium for your bones. This is critical for people over fifty, especially women, in order to prevent osteoporosis. A shortage of vitamin D can also bring on aches and pains similar to symptoms of arthritis.

Again, the G.I. Diet, with its emphasis on low-fat milk and fish, will help, but it won't hurt to top up with a multivitamin, which normally contains the recommended daily level of 400 IU.

Dear Rick,
By following your eating program and walking for 30 minutes at least five times a week I have lost 20 pounds and counting . . . My father was told he had to reduce his cholesterol and had a scare with prostate cancer all in one visit to the doctor! He's been following the G.I. Diet fairly religiously and at 59 years of age, he is back to his college weight!
Jocelyn

Vitamin E

This became the wonder vitamin of the 1990s when it was suggested that it could reduce heart disease, Alzheimer's and certain cancers. There are many significant population studies currently underway, though recent heart disease reports have been somewhat contradictory.

Vitamin E is the one principal vitamin that is underrepresented in most multivitamins. The recommended daily dosage is 100 to 400 IU, whereas most multivitamins contain only 30 to 50 IU. The G.I. Diet will give you a good natural supply of vitamin E, which is found in vegetable oils and nuts (both also sources of "good" fat). However, you would require a significant intake of these vegetable fats to realize the recommended levels. Taking a 400 IU vitamin E supplement is therefore a good idea and carries little risk. Many cardiologists take this supplement, which is as good a recommendation as any.

Fish Oil

There is one oil in particular that has been found to have significant positive health benefits, particularly for your heart. The oil is called omega-3, and it is a fatty acid found primarily in coldwater fish, salmon in particular, as well as in canola and flax seed. As most of us are unlikely to consume salmon on a daily basis, salmon oil is available in capsule form in any pharmacy. I take a couple at breakfast (2000 mg) every day. The research evidence supporting omega-3 is overwhelming and much of it is Canadian, stemming from studies of the Inuit, who do not eat what we consider a heart-healthy diet, with loads of animal fat and virtually no fruit or vegetables. However, the coldwater fish they consume, rich in omega-3, appears to give them protection against heart disease.

TO SUM UP:

The G.I. Diet almost certainly contains sufficient vitamins to meet your daily needs. However, if you are at all concerned, a one-a-day multivitamin offers cheap and risk-free insurance. An extra vitamin E pill is optional, but keep your ears and eyes open to new research on this front. If heart health is a particular concern, omega-3 oil capsules are a good idea. If you are over fifty, particularly if you are female, an extra vitamin D supplement is probably worthwhile.

Appendix I

G.I. Diet Shopping List

PANTRY	FRIDGE/FREEZER
BAKING/COOKING	**DAIRY**
Baking powder/soda	Buttermilk
Cocoa	Cottage cheese (1%)
Dried apricots*	Ice cream (low fat, no added sugar)
Sliced almonds	Milk (skim)
Wheat/oat bran	Sour cream (fat-free or 1%)
Whole wheat flour	Soy milk (plain, low-fat)
BEANS (CANNED)	Yogurt (nonfat with sugar substitute)
Baked beans (low-fat)	**FRUIT**
Mixed salad beans	Apples
Most varieties	Blackberries
Vegetarian chili	Blueberries
BREAD	Cherries
100% stone-ground whole wheat	Grapefruit
CEREALS	Grapes
All-Bran	Lemons
Bran Buds	Limes
Fibre First	Oranges
Kashi Go Lean	Peaches

Oat bran	Pears
Oatmeal (old-fashioned rolled oats)	Plums
	Raspberries
DRINKS	Strawberries
bottled water	**MEAT/POULTRY/FISH/EGGS**
Club soda	All fish and seafood (no breading)
Decaffeinated coffee	Chicken/Turkey breast (skinless)
Diet soft drinks	Extra-lean ground beef
Tea	Lean deli style ham/turkey/chicken
FATS/OILS	Liquid eggs (Break Free/Omega Pro)
Almonds	Pork tenderloin
Canola oil	Veal
Margarine (nonhydrogenated, light)	**VEGETABLES**
Mayonnaise (fat free)	Asparagus
Olive oil	Beans (green/wax)
Salad dressings (fat free)	Bell and hot peppers
Vegetable oil spray	Broccoli
FRUIT (CANNED/BOTTLED)	Cabbage
Applesauce (no sugar)	Carrots
Mandarin oranges	Cauliflower
Peaches in juice or water	Celery
Pears in juice or water	Cucumber
PASTA	Eggplant
Capellini	Leeks
Fettuccine	Lettuce
Macaroni	Mushrooms
Penne	Olives
Spaghetti	Onions
Vermicelli	Pickles
PASTA SAUCES	Potatoes (small, new only)
(vegetable-based only)	Snow peas
Healthy Choice	Spinach
Too Good To Be True	Tomatoes
RICE	Zucchini
Basmati/long grain/wild	**SOUPS**
SEASONINGS	Healthy Choice
Flavoured vinegars/sauces	Too Good To Be True
Spices/herbs	**SWEETENERS**
SNACKS	Equal, Splenda, Sweet'n Low,
Food bars (Zone/Balance)	Sugar Twin (and other
	sugar substitutes)

Appendix II

G.I. Diet Dining Out & Travel Tips

BREAKFAST GREEN LIGHT	BREAKFAST RED LIGHT
Oatmeal	Cold cereals
All-Bran	Muffins
Fruit	Whole regular eggs
Yogurt (nonfat with sugar substitute)	Bacon/sausage
Egg Whites—Omelette	Pancakes/waffles
Egg Whites—Scrambled	
LUNCH GREEN LIGHT	**LUNCH RED LIGHT**
Sandwiches —open-faced/ whole wheat	Potatoes (replace with double vegetables)
Meats—deli style ham/chicken/ turkey	Pasta-based meals
Salads—low fat (dressing on the side)	Fast food
Soups—chunky vegetable-bean	Pizza/white bread/bagels
Wraps—½ pita, no mayonnaise	Cheese
Pasta—¼ plate maximum	Butter/mayonnaise
Vegetables	Baked goods

DINNER GREEN LIGHT	DINNER RED LIGHT
Soups—chunky vegetable and bean	Soups—cream based
Vegetables	Caesar salad
Chicken/turkey (no skin)	Beef/lamb/pork
Fish—not breaded or battered	Potatoes (replace with double vegetables)
Salads—low fat (dressing on the side)	Desserts
Pasta—¼ plate	Bread
Rice (basmati, brown, wild, long grain)—¼ plate	Butter/mayonnaise
Fruit	

SNACKS GREEN LIGHT	SNACKS RED LIGHT
Fresh fruit	Chips, all types
Yogurt—(nonfat with sugar substitute)	Cookies
½ food bar (e.g. Balance)	Muffins
Almonds	Popcorn, regular
Hazelnuts	

PORTIONS	
Meat	Palm of hand / Pack of cards
Vegetables	Minimum ½ plate
Rice/pasta	Maximum ¼ plate

Appendix III

Exercise Calorie Counter

WEIGHT (IN LB):	130	160	200
TIME (IN MIN):	30	30	30
GYM AND HOME ACTIVITIES			
Aerobics: low impact	172	211	264
Aerobics: high impact	218	269	336
Aerobics, Step: low impact	218	269	336
Aerobics, Step: high impact	312	384	480
Aerobics: water	125	154	192
Bicycling, Stationary: moderate	218	269	336
Bicycling, Stationary: vigorous	328	403	504
Circuit Training: general	250	307	384
Rowing, Stationary: moderate	218	269	336
Rowing, Stationary: vigorous	265	326	408
Ski Machine: general	296	365	456
Stair Step Machine: general	187	230	288
Weightlifting: general	94	115	144
Weightlifting: vigorous	187	230	288

TRAINING ACTIVITIES

Basketball: playing a game	250	307	384
Basketball: wheelchair	203	250	312
Bicycling: BMX or mountain	265	326	408
Bicycling: 12–13.9 mph	250	307	384
Bicycling: 14–15.9 mph	312	384	480
Boxing: sparring	281	346	432
Football: competitive	281	346	432
Football: touch, flag, general	250	307	384
Frisbee	94	115	144
Golf: carrying clubs	172	211	264
Golf: using cart	109	134	168
Gymnastics: general	125	154	192
Handball: general	374	461	576
Hiking: cross-country	187	230	288
Horseback Riding: general	125	154	192
Ice Skating: general	218	269	336
Martial Arts: general	312	384	480
Racquetball: competitive	312	384	480
Racquetball: casual, general	218	269	336
Rock Climbing: ascending	343	422	528
Rock Climbing: repelling	250	307	384
Rollerblading	218	269	336
Rope Jumping	312	384	480
Running: 5 mph (12 min/mile)	250	307	384
Running: 5.2 mph (11.5 min/mile)	281	346	432
Running: 6 mph (10 min/mile)	312	384	480
Running: 6.7 mph (9 min/mile)	343	422	528

Running: 7.5 mph (8 min/mile)	390	480	600
Running: 8.6 mph (7 min/mile)	452	557	696
Running: 10 mph (6 min/mile)	515	634	792
Running: pushing wheelchair, marathon wheeling	250	307	384
Running: cross-country	281	346	432
Skiing: cross-country	250	307	384
Skiing: downhill	187	230	288
Snowshoeing	250	307	384
Softball: general play	156	192	240
Swimming: general	187	230	288
Tennis: general	218	269	336
Volleyball: non-competitive, general play	94	115	144
Volleyball: competitive, gymnasium play	125	154	192
Volleyball: beach	250	307	384
Walk: 3.5 mph (17 min/mile)	125	154	192
Walk: 4 mph (15 min/mile)	140	173	216
Walk: 4.5 mph (13 min/mile)	156	192	240
Walk/Jog: jog more than 10 min.	187	230	288
Water Polo	312	384	480
Waterskiing	187	230	288
Whitewater: rafting, kayaking	156	192	240
DAILY LIFE ACTIVITIES			
Children's Games: 4-square, etc.	156	192	240
Chopping & Splitting Wood	187	230	288
Gardening: general	140	173	216
Housecleaning: general	109	134	168
Mowing Lawn: push, hand	172	211	264
Mowing Lawn: push, power	140	173	216

Operate Snow Blower: walking	140	173	216
Raking Lawn	125	154	192
Sex: moderate effort	47	58	72
Shovelling Snow: by hand	187	230	288

Appendix IV

The Ten Golden G.I. Diet Rules

1. Eat three meals and three snacks every day. Don't skip meals—particularly breakfast.

2. Stick with green-light products only in Phase I.

3. When it comes to food, quantity is as important as quality. Shrink your usual portions, particularly of meat, pasta and rice.

4. Always ensure that each meal contains the appropriate measure of carbohydrates, protein and fat.

5. Eat at least three times more vegetables and fruit than usual.

6. Drink plenty of fluids, preferably water.

7. Exercise for thirty minutes once a day or fifteen minutes twice a day. Get off the bus three stops early.

8. Find a friend to join you for mutual support.

9. Set realistic goals. Try to lose an average of a pound a week and record your progress to reinforce your sense of achievement.

10. Don't view this as a diet. It's the basis of how you will eat for the rest of your life.

GIDiet.com

I'm most interested in your feedback on the G.I. Diet. I would particularly like to hear about your personal experience with the diet and any suggestions you might be willing to share. You can contact me at **www.gidiet.com**.

You can also subscribe to the free newsletter, which gives the latest nutritional and medical updates and reader feedback.

G.I. DIET WEEKLY WEIGHT/WAIST LOG

Week	Date	Weight	Waist	Comments
1.				
2.				
3.				
4.				
5.				
6.				
7.				
8.				
9.				
10.				
11.				
12.				
13.				
14.				
15.				
16.				
17.				
18.				
19.				
20.				

G.I. DIET EXERCISE LOG

T = Time   D = Distance

Date	Walking		Jogging		Bicycling		Resistance	Stretching	Other
	T	D	T	D	T	D	repetitions		

Acknowledgements

My thanks and deep appreciation to my friends at Random House Canada who took a flyer on a couple of relative unknowns, myself and the glycemic index, a couple of years ago. I am particularly appreciative of the counsel and wise advice from Anne Collins and for the warm and patient editing of Stacey Cameron. Thanks go to Jennifer Shepherd, who masterminded the selling of international rights in eleven countries around the world, and to Cathy Paine, who has been invaluable in helping bring *The G.I. Diet* to the Canadian public.

To my cheerleader, business adviser and agent, Bruce Westwood, who along with his additional right hand, Natasha Daneman, have been invaluable in extending the G.I. Diet program.

Finally to my wife and partner, Dr. Ruth Gallop, whose insight into women and family needs has added a valuable dimension to the book. Also for her encouragement and support, without which I doubt if *The G.I. Diet* would have seen the light of day.

Index

A

alcohol
    beer, 113
    benefits of, 112
    and blood sugar level, 68
    and weight loss, 68
    wine, 63, 112–13
All-Bran cereal, 15, 36, 88, 172, 174, 230
almonds, 7, 77, 184, 186, 190, 228, 231
    as cereal and fruit topping, 80, 86, 87, 88, 107
    charts, 38, 44, 54
Alzheimer's disease, 6, 216, 222
amino acids, 21
amylose (starch), 56
anchovy fillets, 130, 134, 135
antioxidants, 10, 67
apple juice (unsweetened), 37, 176, 228
apples, 174, 186, 228
    charts, 37, 43, 53
    as dessert or snack, 77
    and glycemic index, 15, 17–18

applesauce
    with sugar, 37
    unsweetened, 57, 77, 81, 86, 174, 176, 229
apricots, 37, 43, 53, 176
artichokes, 43
artificial sweeteners. *See* sugar substitutes
arugula, 43, 53
asparagus, 43, 53, 94, 103, 229
avocado, 43, 63

B

backpack motivator, 70–71, 114
baked beans, 78, 164, 228
bacon
    back, 36, 41, 90, 120
    regular, 36, 41, 42, 230
    turkey, 36, 41, 229, 230
Baechle, Thomas, 214
bagels, 11, 15, 37, 43, 53, 230
baguette, 15, 37, 43, 53
Balance Bar, 50

bananas
    charts, 37, 43, 53
    as dessert, 57
    and insulin levels, 31
barbecuing, 86
barley, 14, 77
beans, 90, 92, 102, 116, 126, 132, 134, 158, 164. *See also* baked beans; *specific beans*
    charts, 43, 53
    and glycemic index, 15, 77
    and protein and fibre, 14, 20–21, 77
    and vegetarian diet, 64
beef. *See also* ground beef
    lean cuts, 42, 52, 103
    steaks, 5, 55, 103, 168
beer, 113
beets, 43, 53
berries, 37, 57. *See also specific berries*
beverages, 35, 65–68. *See also specific beverages*
black beans, 116, 118
blackberries, 44, 54
blood sugar levels, 16, 68, 75
blueberries, 173, 178, 186, 188, 194, 228
BMI. *See* Body Mass Index
body fat, 23, 24
    abdominal, 25, 222
Body Mass Index (BMI), 23–24, 26–27, 30, 32
body weight measurements
    BMI, 23–24, 26–27, 30, 32
    waist circumference, iv, 24–25
bone density, 225
Bran Buds cereal, 36, 88, 174, 228
breads
    "brown," 12
    charts, 37, 43, 53
    and food pyramids, 59, 60
    and grain processing, 12, 13, 40

    and insoluble fibre, 14
    pita, 43, 49, 230
    in sandwiches, 45
    serving sizes, 63, 78
    stone-ground whole wheat, 40, 43, 53, 78, 96, 146
    white, 12, 37, 51, 230
    whole-grain, 37, 43, 53
breakfast, 86–91, 116–22, 186
    charts, 36–38
    in Phase I, 38–41
    in Phase II, 110
    and protein, 21
    skipping, 35
Bregman, Michael, 11
broad beans, 31, 43, 53
broccoli, 44, 54, 90, 94, 98, 102, 146, 229
brunch, 118, 146, 148
Brussels sprouts, 44, 54
bulgur, 136
butter, 6, 8, 38, 41, 44, 54
buttermilk, 36, 228

C
cabbage, 44, 54, 229
Caesar salads, 48, 134
caffeine, 66, 67, 69
calcium, 225
calorie counter (exercise), 232–35
calories
    and energy, 17, 28
    and exercise, 205–06
    and fat, v, 5, 19, 205
    and labels, 73
    and protein, 19
    source of, 28–29
    and weight gain, 4
Canada's Food Guide, 10
Canadian diet, current, 8–9
cancer, 6, 10, 25, 221
candy, 51, 62

canola
    oil, 7, 38, 44, 54, 63, 229
    seed, 7
capellini, 229
carbohydrates
    charts, 36, 43, 53
    and diabetes, 221
    and fast food, 62
    and food pyramids, 59, 60
    as part of healthy diet, 3, 10,
        13–14, 28, 29
    and weight loss, 10
carrots, 44, 54, 98, 100, 142, 229
cauliflower, 44, 54, 98, 124, 229
celery, 44, 54, 229
cereals, 6, 8, 14. *See also specific*
  breakfast cereals
    chart, 36
    cold, 13, 39, 79
    on food pyramids, 58–60
    and glycemic index, 15
    and grain processing, 12
    serving sizes, 73
Cheerios cereal, 15
cheese
    charts, 36, 42
    to enhance flavour, 86
    fat-free, 40, 42, 52
    feta, 40, 138, 142
    low-fat, 20, 42, 52, 144
    regular, 40, 42, 52. 230
    and saturated fat, 6, 40, 47
    skim milk, 90
    Stilton, 40
cheesecake, 188
cherries, 37, 44, 54, 228
chicken, 94, 126, 154, 160
    breast (skinless), 42, 52, 55,
        97–100, 151, 229
    ground, 162
    thighs (skinless), 156

chickpeas, 116, 124, 130, 136, 142,
    148, 150, 156, 162
children, and G.I. diet, 63–64
Chinese food, 49
chocolate, 183, 184
    dark, 112
    serving size, 63, 112
cholesterol, 6, 41, 73, 86
    and fibre, 14
    HDL (good), 219
    and heart disease, 6, 7, 39, 81,
        113, 218, 219
    LDL (bad), 77, 219
    and oatmeal, 39, 81
club soda, 229
coconut oil, 6
coffee, 21, 41, 66, 110
    decaffeinated, 41, 66–67
cookies, 180–85
    charts, 37, 43, 51, 53
    as snack, 12, 16, 50, 51, 107
cooking tips, 85–86, 88
corn, 12, 31, 44, 53, 111
cornflakes, 15
corn oil, 7, 8, 54
cottage cheese, 95, 142, 188
    low-fat, 20
    1% or fat-free, 36, 40, 42, 53, 79,
        228
    as snack, 50, 79, 107
    whole or 2%, 36, 42, 53
crab, 148
crackers, 8, 12
cranberries, 37
cream, 36
    substitutes for, 86
cream cheese, 42
    light, 36, 42, 118, 188
crispbreads, 37, 43, 63
croissants, 37, 43, 53
croutons, 43
cucumbers, 44, 54, 132, 229

D

dairy products, 10, 40, 57
    and protein, 20
    charts, 36, 42, 52
    and food pyramids, 59, 60
dessert, 47, 57, 180–94
    low-G.I. alternatives, 57
diabetes
    diet and, 216, 220–21
    exercise and, 201, 220
    and hypoglycemia, 38
    risk factors for, 25, 220
    Type 2, 220, 222
diets, viii, ix, 1, 2, 10
digestive system, 5, 10, 13, 14, 16–17,
    18, 21, 35, 65, 66
dining out, 46, 241
dinner, 21
    charts, 52–55
    meal ideas, 97–106
    in Phase I, 55–57
    in Phase II, 111
    portion ratios, 58
donuts, 15, 37, 43, 53
dried fruit, 37, 43, 53, 173
Dynaband, 214

E

eggplant, 44, 54, 142, 144, 229
eggs, 89, 116, 118, 120, 130, 192
    charts, 36, 42, 52
    and cholesterol, 40–41
    and food pyramids, 59, 60
    low-cholesterol liquid, 20,
        40–41, 79
    omega-3, 79
energy
    and carbohydrates and glucose,
        10, 15, 16
    and exercise, 71, 205
    from fat cells, 25, 28
    in Phase I and Phase II, 108–09

Equal, 83, 88, 229
exercise
    benefits of, 200, 201
    bicycling, 202, 207, 210
    and calorie consumption,
        205–06, 212
    calorie counter, 232-235
    equipment, 202, 203, 211–13
    excuses not to, 201–04
    hiking, 209
    indoor, 202–03, 211–13
    jogging, 202, 207, 209
    log, 207, 241
    outdoor sports, 202, 210
    in Phase I and Phase II, 200
    and protein, 29, 206
    resistance exercises, 206–07
    resistance training, 213–14
    stretching, 214–15
    walking, 202, 205–06, 207, 208
    for weight maintenance, v, 200,
        204–07, 212

F

fast food, 47–49. *See also specific foods*
    and energy, 16
    and fat, 47
    and serving sizes, 62
fats
    calorie content, 5
    charts, 38, 44, 54
    comparison of, 5–6
    cooking with, 85–86
    and digestion, 5, 18–19
    and fast food, 8, 47
    and food pyramids, 59, 60
    and glucose, 18
    hydrogenated, 6
    and labels, 8, 73
    monounsaturated ("best"), 7,
        219
    polyunsaturated, 7, 219

saturated ("bad"), 5–6, 219, 221, 222
fettuccine, 15, 31, 43, 53, 168, 229
fibre, 14
  and beans, 20–21
  and breads, 40
  and cold cereals, 39
  and digestion, 14
  and labels, 39, 73
  in "slow release" foods, 14
Fibre First cereal, 36, 228
fish, 101, 150–53, 150, 152
  benefits of, 55, 79
  breaded or coated, 20, 42, 52, 55, 79
  charts, 42, 52
  and food pyramids, 59, 60
  serving size, 56, 63
  and vitamin D, 225
fish oil, 7
flavonoids, 67, 112
flax seed, 7
flour, 12–13, 62, 78
  partial substitute for, 81
folic acid, 224
food bars, 50, 51, 79–80, 107
food charts
  breakfast, 36–38
  dinner, 52–55
  fats, 8
  G.I. ratings (sample), 15
  grain consumption, 11
  lunch, 42–45
  snacks, 51
food guide, 10
Food Pyramid (G.I.), 60
Food Pyramid (USDA), 59
fructose, 83
fruitcake, 18
fruit cocktail, 37
fruit drinks, 37, 68
fruit juices, 37, 38, 68

fruits, 87, 88, 95, 186, 188, 192. See
  also specific fruits
  better than fruit juices, 38
  charts, 37, 43, 51, 53, 228, 231
  as dessert, 47, 57
  dried, 37, 43, 53, 173
  fibre and citrus, 14
  and food pyramids, 59, 60
  fresh, 37, 64, 89, 224
  as snacks, 50, 51, 107
fruit spreads, 41

G
garlic, 134, 158
G.I. Diet
  and children, 63–64
  colour-coded food charts, 36–38, 42–45, 51, 52–55
  diet chart, 33–34
  dining out and travel tips, 230–31
  exercise log, 241
  "falling off the wagon," 74, 114
  food pyramid, 60, 61
  newsletter, 76
  Phase I and Phase II compared, 29–31, 108–09
  portions, 58
  research on effectiveness of, 3
  sample G.I. ratings, 15
  shopping list, 228–29
  Ten Rules, 236–37
  weekly weight/waist log, 71–72, 75, 239
gidiet.com, 3, 238
ginger, 86
glucose, 10, 15–17, 238. See also sugar
glycemic index, 15–19
grains
  charts, 37, 43, 53
  and food pyramids, 59, 60
  as part of high-carbohydrate diet, 10–11

and processing, 12, 13
granola, 36, *186*
granola bars
    homemade, 37, 50, 51, *176*
grapefruit, 15, 37, 44, 54, 80, 228
grapefruit juice (unsweetened), 37
grapes, 31, 37, 44, 54, 228
green beans, 43, 53, *102*, *130*, *156*, 229
green-light ("go ahead") foods, 31, 35, 77–84
Green-Light Menu Plan, 195–99
grilling, 86
ground beef, *104*, *106*, *166*, *170*
    alternatives to, 106
    extra-lean, 42, 52, 229
    lean, 42, 52
    regular, 42, 52

H
ham (lean), 36, 42, 52, *103*, *120*, *164*, 229
hamburger buns, 43
hamburgers, 42, 47, 48, 52, 80
Harvard School of Public Health study, 29
hash browns, 38
hazelnuts, 38, 51, 54, 231
Healthy Weight Pyramid (Mayo Clinic), 58
heart disease, 217–18
    and alcohol, 112
    and antioxidants, 10, 67
    and cholesterol, 6, 7, 39, 81, 113, 218, 219
    and diet, 55, 216, 218
    and exercise, 201, 207
    and fats, viii, 6
    and risk factors, 25
    and vitamin E, 226
herbs and spices, 231
homocysteine, 224

hot dog buns, 43
hot dogs, 42, 52
hummus, 45, 96
hunger
    and caffeine, 66
    and calories, 28
    and dieting, 2
    and protein, 20
    and snacks, 20
hydrogenated oils, 6
hypertension (high blood pressure), 218–19
hypoglycemia (low blood sugar), 38

I
ice cream
    low-fat, 42, 51
    —— and sugar-free, 42, 51, 57, 80
    regular, 51, 237
insulin, 16–17

J
juices. *See* fruit juices; vegetable juices

K
Kashi Go Lean cereal, 36, 228
Kashi Good Friends cereal, 36
kidney beans, 15, 16, *140*, *160*
    red, *104*, *118*, *138*, *158*, *166*
    white, *104*, *122*, *141*, *183*
kiwi fruit, 37, 44, 54

L
labels on food, 8, 73
lamb, 231
    lean cuts, 42, 52, *151*
leeks, 44, 54
legumes. *See* beans
lemons, 44, 54, 233
lettuce, 43, 53, *128*, *130*, *134*, 229

lima beans, 156
limes, 132
linguine, 43, 53
low-carb diet, 10
lunch, 92–96
    charts, 42–45
    meal ideas, 45–47
    in Phase I, 45–49
    in Phase II, 110
    and protein, 21
    recipes, 92–96

M

macaroni, 43, 53, 229
    and cheese, 43, 53, 144
mandarin oranges, 152
mangoes, 37, 44, 54
margarine
    hard, 38, 44, 54
    nonhydrogenated, 38, 44, 54
    nonhydrogenated, light, 38, 41,
        44, 55, 229
    serving sizes, 63
    soft (tub), 38, 41, 44, 54, 55
Mayo Clinic Healthy Weight
    Pyramid, 58
mayonnaise
    fat-free, 44, 54, 86
    light, 44, 54
    regular, 44, 54
McDonald's, 47, 48
meat. *See also specific meats*
    charts, 36, 42, 52
    and fats, 6, 20, 55, 103
    and food pyramids, 59, 60
    grilling and barbecuing, 86
    and protein, 20
    serving size, 56, 63, 103
meatless recipes, 136–47
Mediterranean diet, 7
melba toast, 18, 31

melons, 37, 43, 53. *See also specific
    melons*
menopause and alcohol, 113
menu plan, 195–99
meringues, 192
metabolism, 206
Mexican food, 49
milk
    1%, 36, 39, 53
    skim, 18, 20, 36, 39, 42, 66, 80,
        228
    2%, 39, 42, 53
    and vitamin D, 225
    whole, 18, 42, 53
milkshakes, 48
motivation tips, 70–72, 74–76, 114
muesli, 31, 36, 87
muffins, 11, 15, 172, 174
    charts, 37, 43, 51, 53, 230, 231
    as snacks, 50
multivitamins, 224, 225, 226, 227
muscle mass, 206, 213
mushrooms, 43, 53, 140, 170, 229
mussels, 156
mustard, 45, 96, 128, 130

N

navy beans, 164
noodles, 15–16
    canned or instant, 43, 53
nut butters, 38
nuts. *See also specific nuts*
    charts, 38, 44, 54
    and food pyramids, 59, 60
    and protein, 21
    serving sizes, 63
    as snacks, 107
    as source of "good" fat, 80
    and vitamin E, 226

O

oat bran, 36, 39, 79, 81, 174, 229
oatmeal, 81, 87, 230
   and cholesterol, 39, 81
   and fibre, 14
   and glycemic index, 15, 86
   as "slow-release" food, 13, 86
   as snack, 81
oats, old-fashioned rolled, 39, 79,
   81, 86, 176, 177, 178, 180, 182, 186
obesity, viii
   in adults, 4
   and carbohydrates, 9, 58
   in children, 4, 64
   and diabetes, 220
   and fats, 8–9
   and high blood pressure, 218–19
oils. *See also* fats; *specific oils*
   comparison chart, 8
   fish, 7, 227
   and food pyramids, 59, 60
   hydrogenated, 6
   monounsaturated ("best"), 7
   polyunsaturated ("better"), 7
   tropical, 6, 38, 55
   vegetable, 6, 7, 38, 55
   and vitamin E, 226
olive oil
   charts, 38, 44, 54
   as cooking oil, 7
   serving size, 63
olives, 7, 43, 53, 63, 229
omega-3, 7, 79, 227
   eggs, 36, 42, 52, 79
100% Bran cereal, 230
onions, 43, 53, 229
oranges, 15, 37, 43, 54, 81, 228
   mandarin, 152
orange juice (unsweetened), 37, 38,
   81
osteoporosis, 201, 225

P

palm oil, 6
pancakes, 37, 43, 230
papayas, 37, 44, 54
parsnips, 43
pasta, 94, 168, 170. *See also* specific
   pastas
   alfredo, 46
   average consumption of, 12
   and carbohydrates, 10
   charts, 43, 53
   cooking *al dente*, 81
   in food pyramids, 59, 60
   and glycemic index, 46
   and obesity, 46
   serving size, 46, 56, 63, 81, 102
   whole grain, 46, 56, 81
pasta sauces, 46, 163, 229
paté, 42
peaches, 37, 44, 54, 81, 228
   canned, 81
peanut butter, 18, 38, 44, 54, 182
peanuts, 7, 182
pear juice (unsweetened), 37
pears, 44, 54, 81, 172, 190, 229
   canned, 81
peas, 44, 54, 136, 156
penne, 43, 53, 229
peppers
   bell, 43, 54
   green bell, 132, 160, 170
   hot, 44, 54, 132
   orange bell, 168
   red bell, 168, 170
   roasted red, 146
pickles, 44, 51, 54, 229
pineapples, 37, 44, 54
pita bread, 43, 49, 53, 166, 230
pizza, 43, 49, 53, 138, 230
plums, 37, 44, 54, 229
pomegranates, 54
popcorn, 15, 51, 62, 111, 236, 231

pork, *132*, 229, 231
  lean cuts, 42, 52
porridge. *See* oatmeal
portions, 58
potato chips, 51, 231
potatoes
  baked, 15, 44, 54, 82
  boiled, 44, 46, 54
  boiled new, 44, 54, 56, 82, *102*, 130, 136
  french fries, 38, 43, 48, 51, 53
  fried, 82
  and glycemic index, 56
  mashed, 44, 54, 82
  serving size, 56, 63, 82
  and starch, 82
poultry, 20, 63, *97–100*, *154–61*. *See also* chicken; turkey
pretzels, 51
processed meats, 42, 52
processing of food, 12, 13
protein
  as brain food, 21
  charts, 36, 42, 52
  and digestion, 18
  and exercise, 29
  and fat, 20
  and food pyramids, 59, 60
  and lunches, 45
  sources of low-fat, 20–21
prune juice, 37
pudding, 51
pumpkin seeds, 51

R
radishes, 44, 54
raisins, 15, 51, *186*
raspberries, 44, 54, *188*, 229
recipes. *See* Recipe Index
red-light ("stop") foods, 31
Red River cereal, 36
red wine, 63

resistance training, 213–14
rice, *94*, *128*, *156*, *160*
  basmati, 31, 43, 47, 53, 56, 82, 102, *156*, 229, 231
  brown, 43, 47, 53, 56, 82, *128*, *160*, 231
  charts, 43, 53
  and food pyramids, 59, 60
  glutinous, 47, 49, 82
  and glycemic index, 15–16, 56, 82
  instant, 15, 43, 53
  long-grain, 43, 47, 53, 56, 82, 229, 231
  serving size, 47, 56, 63
  short-grain, 43, 53
  white, 43, 53
  wild, 43, 53, 56, 229, 231
rice cakes, 31, 51
rutabaga, 44

S
salads, 45, 57, 82, *92–94*, *128–34*
  fast food, 48
  and protein, 45
salad dressings, *128*, *130*, *132*, *134*
  fat-free, 44, 55, 57
  light, 44, 45, 54, 57, 230, 231
  regular, 44, 54
  vinaigrette, 82
salmon, 55, 79, 96, *101*
salsa, 86
salt, 49
sandwiches, *154*
  alternatives for spreads, 45, 96
  chicken or tuna salad, 96
  and glycemic index, 45
  rules for, 45, 96
sauces, 229
  cheese, *142*, *144*
  pasta, 46, *163*, 229
sausages, 36, 42, 52

seafood, 42, 52, 148, 156
seasonings, 229
serving sizes, 58, 61–63
    and labels, 73
    in Phase II, 109–11
shopping list, 228–29
shopping tips, 72–74
shortening, 38, 55
Shredded Wheat cereal, 36
shrimp, 134, 148, 156, 161
side dishes, 102
sleep, 204
"slow-release" foods, 13, 14, 86
smoking, 217
snacks, 172–79, 186
    and carbohydrates, 10, 11
    charts, 51, 236
    and fats, 6, 8, 107
    in Phase I, 50
    in Phase II, 111
    as sugar fix, 16
    suggestions for, 107, 111
snow peas, 44, 54, 168, 229
soft drinks
    caffeine-free, 66
    diet, 66
    and sugar, 66
sorbet, 51
soups, 82, 122–27 , 229, 230, 231
    charts, 45, 51, 55
    homemade with green-light
        ingredients, 51, 55, 82
sour cream
    alternative to, 105
    light, 36, 53, 83, 228
    regular, 36, 53
soy products
    protein powder, 83
    soy cheese, 232
    soy milk, 36, 53, 80, 83, 228
    tofu, 42, 83
    spaghetti, 15, 43, 53, 162, 229

spinach, 44, 54, 120, 122, 128, 141, 158,
    229
Splenda, 83, 88, 229
spreads. *See* fruit spreads; margarine
squash, 44, 54
steak, 5, 55, 103, 168
strawberries, 44, 54, 186, 188, 229
Strength Training Past 50, 214
stretching, 214–15
stroke
    and alcohol, 112
    and diet, 216, 217
    and exercise, 201, 207
submarines, 48
Subway, 48
sugar. *See also* glucose; sugar
    substitutes
    and beverages, 35, 66
    and digestion, 15
    and glycemic index, 15, 16
sugar substitutes, 35, 39–40, 83, 229
    cooking with, 88
Sugar Twin, 83, 88, 229
sunflower
    seeds, 51, 176, 186
    oil, 7, 233
supplements, 223. *See also individual
    vitamins*
sushi, 52
sweeteners. *See* sugar substitutes
Sweet'N Low, 83, 229
sweet potatoes, 44, 54

T
tea, 67, 229
Thera-Band, 214
"thrift gene," 220
tofu, 42, 83
tomatoes
    canned, 116, 142, 156, 164, 166,
        170
    charts, 44, 54

and glycemic index, 15
fresh, *128, 130, 132, 134, 146, 150, 160*
tortellini, 43, 53
tortilla chips, 51
tortillas, 53, *116*
trail mix, 51
trans fat, 6
tropical oils, 6, 38, 44
trout, *101*
tuna, 86, *130, 150*
turkey
    bacon, 42. 230
    breast (skinless), 42, 52, 55, *158, 161,* 229
    ground, *162*

U
USDA Food Pyramid, 58, 59

V
veal, *103, 170, 235*
vegetables. *See also specific vegetables*
    as backbone of dinner, 57
    charts, 38, 43, 51
    and food pyramids, 59, 60
    frozen, 57
    raw, 50
    serving size, 57
    as snack, 50, 51
vegetable oils, 6, 7, 86
vegetable oil sprays, 85–86, 229
vegetable shortening, 38
vegetarian recipes, *136–46, 167*
vegetarians, 64–65
vermicelli, 43, 53, 229
vinegar, 229
Vitamin B, 224
Vitamin C, 224
Vitamin D, 225
Vitamin E, 226

W
waffles, 37, 43, 230
waist circumference, iv, 24–25
walnuts, 55
water, 66, 229
watermelon juice, 37
weight loss target, 32
weight measurement, 23–27
Westcott, Wayne, 214
wheat bran, 88, *172, 176, 177, 178, 180, 182, 186*
wheat germ, *186*
wine, 63, 112–13
wraps, 48
www.gidiet.com, 3, 238

Y
yams, 44, 54
yellow-light ("caution") foods, 31
yogurt
    added to cereal, 39, 84
    fat- and sugar-free, 15, 20, 36, 39, 47, 57, 230
    fruit (fat- and sugar-free) , 42, 51, 53, 84
    low-fat, 20, 36, 39, 42, 53, *172, 188, 194*
    as snack, 50, 84, *107*
    whole or 2%, 36, 53
yogurt cheese, 84, *105, 190*

Z
Zone Bar, 50
zucchini, 44, 54, *144, 170,* 229

Recipe Index

A
Almond-Crusted Pears, 190
Anchovy Garlic Dressing, 134
Anchovy Mustard Vinaigrette, 130
Apple Bran Muffins, 174
Asian Stir-fry, 98

B
Baked Beans, 164
Basmati Rice Paella, 156
Bean and Onion Pizza, 138
Béchamel Sauce, 170
Blueberry Bars, 178

C
Cauliflower and Chickpea Soup, 124
Cheesecake, Crustless Fruit-topped, 188
Cheese Sauce, 142
Chewy Peanut Bars, 182
Chicken Curry, 100
Chicken, Italian, 99
Chicken Jambalaya, 160
Chili, 104

Chili Lime Vinaigrette, 132
Chocolate Almond Slices, 184
Chocolate Drop Cookies, 183
Classic Meat Lasagna, 170
Cottage Cheese and Fruit, 95
Cream of Spinach Soup, 122
Crustless Fruit-topped Cheesecake, 188

F
Fish: Basic Preparation, 101
Fish Steak with Tomato Chickpea Relish, Quick, 150
Frozen Blueberry Treat, 194
Fruit and Yogurt Parfaits, 186
Fruit-filled Pavlova, 192

G
Greek Salad, 93
Green Eggs and Ham, 120

H
Homemade Granola Bars, 176
Homemade Muesli, 87
Huevos Rancheros, 116

I
Italian Chicken, 99

J
Jerk Pork Salad, 132

L
Lasagna, Classic Meat, 170

M
Macaroni and Cheese, Roasted Vegetable, 144
Mandarin Salsa, 152
Meat Loaf, 106
Mediterranean Rice Salad with Tangy Mustard Herb Dressing, 128
Mixed Bean Salad, 92
Muesli, Homemade, 87
Muffins, Apple Bran, 174
Mushroom and Bean Ragout, 140

N
Niçoise Salad, 130

O
Oatcakes, 177
Oatmeal, 87
Oatmeal Cookies, 180
Omelette and Variations, Basic, 89
On-the-Run Breakfast, 88
Open-Faced Chicken Reuben Sandwich, 154
Over-the-Top Bran Muffins with Pear, 172

P
Pan-Seared White Fish with Mandarin Salsa, 152
Pavlova, Fruit-filled, 192
Pizza, Bean and Onion, 138
Poultry: Basic Preparation, 97

Q
Quick Fish Steak with Tomato Chickpea Relish, 150

R
Roasted Pepper and Tomato Strata, 146
Roasted Vegetable Macaroni and Cheese, 144

S
Sesame Garlic Marinade, 158
Shrimp Caesar Salad, 134
Shrimp and Crab Cakes, 148
Sloppy Joes, 166
Southwest Chicken and Bean Soup, 126
Southwest Omelette Roll-up, 118
Spaghetti and Meatballs, 162
Spinach-Stuffed Turkey Breast, 158
Steak Fettuccine, 168

T
Tangy Mustard Herb Dressing, 128
Tomato Chickpea Relish, 150

V
Vegetarian Moussaka, 142
Vegetarian Shepherd's Pie, 136

W
Waldorf Chicken and Rice Salad, 94
White Bean Mash, 141

NOTES

NOTES

NOTES

NOTES

NOTES